THE
TORTOISE
~~DIET~~ *Method*

Winning the weightloss race –
for those who never want to diet again

KEREN MACKAY

First published by Ultimate World Publishing 2023
Copyright © 2023 Keren Mackay

ISBN

Paperback: 978-1-923123-17-5
Ebook: 978-1-923123-18-2

Cover design: Ultimate World Publishing
Layout and typesetting: Ultimate World Publishing
Editor: Vanessa McKay
Photographer: Penelope Maguire

Ultimate World Publishing
Diamond Creek,
Victoria Australia 3089
www.writeabook.com.au

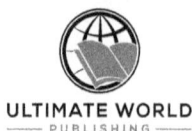

Dedication

For

Penelope and Lily, Aileen and Jasmin

and for

Murray

Without whom none of this would have happened.

Contents

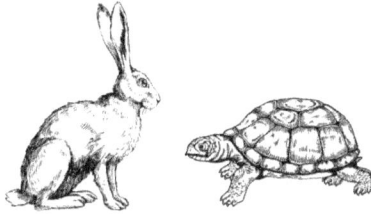

Prologue

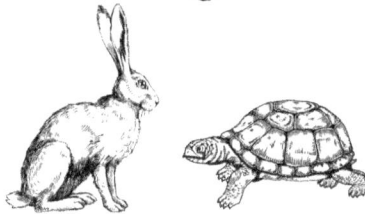

The Hare had been boasting around the village about how fast it was and how it could beat any challengers in a running race. It even started picking on the tortoise – a creature not exactly physically endowed for speed. Finally, the tortoise agreed to the challenge, and a course was duly marked out and a finishing line set up. The hare thought it was a great joke and mockingly showed up at the starting line beside the lumbering tortoise. Off went the starting gun and off went the hare at a great rate of knots until it was a blur in the distance. Meanwhile, the tortoise set off at a slow but steady pace and headed straight towards the finish line.

The hare, full of confidence, looked back and could not even see its opponent. Oh well, he said, might as well stop for a snack and went off and had a few cabbages. A bit later, it got back on track and zoomed off again. Still no sign of the tortoise. So, it stopped again and had a nap. Meanwhile, the tortoise did not stop its steady focused journey and made its way step by step toward that finishing line. Sometime during the day, the tortoise passed by the sleeping hare and as it approached the finishing line, the cheers of the villagers woke the hare. Up jumped the hare in sleepy surprise and took off again as fast as it could, but it was too late.

Slow and steady had won the race!

Introduction

A Love Letter to The Reader

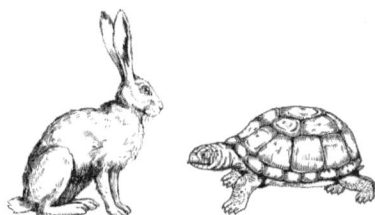

Frankly, I never want to go on a diet ever again. I have given up on them – or maybe they have given up on me. For most of us, the traditional restrictive-eating type of diet simply does not work and in fact seems to end up making us fatter than when we started out. I'm not even sure I was even overweight when I started on my first diet. In fact, I know I wasn't as I have recently found my original weight-loss tracker from the first time I went on a proper official diet, and I can only vaguely recall ever being as tiny as the number on that piece of paper. And I am talking about the starting weight on it – not the goal weight!

Not only have they not worked, but they have kept us in the pain of a self-defeating behavioural loop resulting in a pattern of lifelong failure. And most infuriating of all, the time, energy and emotions wasted, the amount of pain silently suffered in the lives of otherwise intelligent, talented women who could do so much more without this seemingly senseless struggle to be thin.

I may have given up on dieting, but I hadn't given up on looking my best or being happy and healthy – I just figured there must be another way to do it that didn't cost so much in terms of our personal lives or was clearly never going to work. This put me in a bit of a dilemma. So, I did something that I should have done a lot earlier in my life.

You've all heard the adage attributed to Einstein; the definition of crazy is repeating the same behaviour over and again and expecting different results. That is exactly what I was doing - getting sucked into the hope of the next diet being the one that will finally save me but ending up back where I was before I started. We get sucked into every miracle-promising diet that comes our way- which it does regularly if we are looking.

In the interests of moving away from crazy, I had this rather brilliant idea of looking at my own life and the lives of others who had been successful and seeing if there were any lessons to be learned. If success leaves clues, what were they? Instead of embarking on another diet, I started looking at the reasons traditional diets had not worked for me and probably for most of you either. I asked the right questions of myself and came up with some answers that have helped me greatly and I think will help you too.

What had I been doing to put on weight in the first place? What had worked for me in the past when I had achieved good weight loss results, and by the same process, what had not worked? What were the things that stopped me from getting to my end goal and what were the things that helped me when I was successful? I really wanted to understand the whole life wasting exercise that preoccupation with the scales can be.

The book you are holding in your hands today is not a be all and end all book about nutrition, physiology, or human behaviour – nor is it even a book about a diet in the traditional sense of the word. If you are looking for a book that will tell you how to lose 10 kilos by last Friday, then this is not the book for you. What you will find in this book, is a good down to earth look at the life of ordinary people, mainly women, who have struggled for years with traditional dieting but never succeeded in losing or sustaining weight loss for a meaningful length of time, and it asks why. Why have we not only failed to lose weight and keep it off but very often end up putting more on? Why do we do it again and again and what can we do differently that works? The answers to those questions lead me to what you will be reading in this book.

I wrote it because I had to. I was tired of seeing myself and many others around me not living the lives we were meant to live because we felt we had to be a certain weight in order to do so but were then caught in the terrible trap of never being able to succeed in reaching that weight – whatever it was.

I wrote it because after a lifetime of dieting, going up and down in the weight department with my self-esteem matching every rise and fall, I realised I had spent way too much time thinking and worrying about the problem of losing weight when there were a lot more important things I should have been doing. Living the life I was put here on earth to do for example.

I wrote it because of the psychological and emotional cost of being overweight, and the very real health issues it can bring. The older you are, the more likely diet related illnesses show up. Finding a way to send the number on the scales heading downward rather than an increasingly upward trajectory becomes increasingly important.

And I wrote it because I was tired of being a failure. How could I preach and teach when I couldn't even reach the goal myself? I realised I could never become the person I wanted to be unless I overcame that for myself. Losing weight for me represented a major barrier in my life that was much more than just weight loss. I began to lose hope in ever winning the race. What sort of example was I setting to my own daughters? And I don't just mean in losing weight – but in breaking through a personal barrier and getting to the next level. I had always believed we were capable of more – why couldn't I even lose a few pounds and keep them off?

Most of all, I wrote it as a love letter to you. Because I know that many of you have been on the same painful journey as I have, and I feel such compassion for you. I got off that diet treadmill and gently and sensibly broke through that barrier once and for all, and if I can do it, so can you.

I call it the gentle path because the old behaviour of striving and straining to reach what has been quite frankly, an impossible goal, is no longer the path you are going to take. This way will begin where you are right now and gently turn you in the direction you need to go to take the right steps daily to get there.

Following this method will enable you to lose weight. It does this because it takes a long-term approach to a way of living that takes the time to understand the why, how to identify and overcome the obstacles, and then provide you with the tools and strategies to sustain those changes over time, reversing the upward trend showing up on the scales and head you in the right direction on your pathway to finally winning.

To give you a sneak peek - the Tortoise Diet Method is a gentle response to the three questions central to the problem of how to lose weight and keep it off:

- How did I get here in the first place?
- Why have traditional diets not worked for me?
- What do I need to do to finally win this race?

Just a note on the word *diet*. It is potentially an emotional trigger point for some people and therefore not really a useful word to use when thinking of long-term health and well-being. I would like to challenge the diet mindset out there that says there is something wrong with us if we don't fit into a certain mould or look a certain way and we must suffer in order to do that. I would hate to think any young person who is reading this thinks that they have to be thin to be beautiful or acceptable and that the only way to do that is to follow a calorie controlled, restrictive way of eating designed to reduce pleasure, be non-sociable, impossible to maintain and leading to a lifetime of gain. That's what I mean by a traditional diet.

The word should just be a noun; a word describing the food we eat. As in "the tortoise lives on a diet of leafy greens and fruits." So, when I use the "D" word, please remember that I am not referring to restriction for the sake of a short-term goal, but more about how you choose to eat over the course of your daily life that is going to lead to your desired outcome. It's just that it's difficult to write a book about diet without actually using the word! Which is why the word diet is crossed out in the title and the word method is included. You will find that I used both words interchangeably in this book.

7

My biggest hope from this book is that you don't make this just another 'diet' book or another failed quest for success in life. The *Tortoise Diet Method* will work best when you make it your own personal method and adapt it to your age and stage in life. I asked a lot of questions of myself to come up with this method and if you ask the same of yourself, you will get the answers you need as you work your way through the book. Adapt the plan to your life and you will end up with your own personal blueprint for success. I have included some what I call 'success work' at the end of some chapters. Use your own journal to do this work or contact me to get your own printable copy of the *Tortoise Diet Method Workbook*.

You will also see that the book has been structured around the metaphor of the race and as the fable is set in the classical era I've had a bit of fun turning signposts into guideposts and goals into milestones along the road, just as you would have found back then.

I have broken it down into the 5 Stages of a race and included 12 key Guideposts that will guide you along the way as you make the *Tortoise Diet Method* your own. They will be summarised at the end of the book so you can check against your own roadmap.

So, this book is not about a new diet, but it is about taking the age-old wisdom encountered in the age-old tale about the Tortoise and the Hare and applying it to the here and now in our own lives starting today.

Your race starts.... Now!

Stage 1

Life is Like a Race

*If trying to lose weight is like a life race –
I have been losing it!*

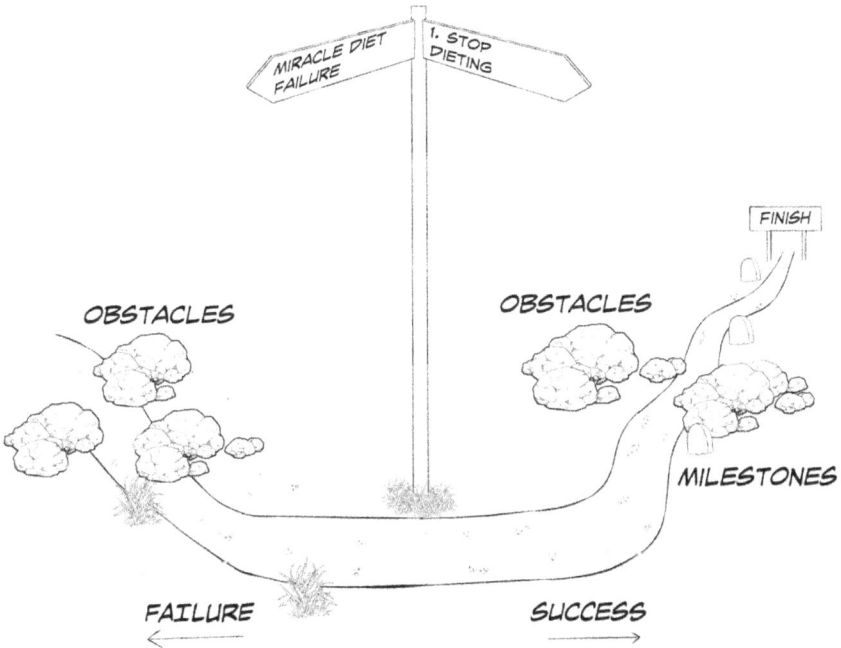

Chapter 1

Life Lessons In Losing

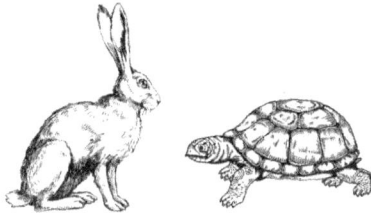

Let me immediately assure you that this diet does not involve eating or otherwise interfering with tortoises in any way, shape, or form. You can rest assured that no tortoises will be harmed by your participation in the Tortoise Diet. The tortoise, in this case, takes its name from the ancient Greek fable by Aesop known as 'The Tortoise and the Hare'.

Aesop, of course, was writing in the Classical Greek era, but obviously nothing about the human condition has changed in the intervening 2500 years or so. In this story, Aesop cleverly uses the metaphor of the Tortoise and the Hare to tell us something about human behaviour. He knew such metaphors can be very helpful in showing us, through the medium of storytelling and imagination, universal truths about the human condition. How we behave and how perhaps we ought to behave. They can provide insight that can lead to self-awareness, which can ultimately lead to changes in behaviour. It is those behavioural changes, which when they become part of your life, will be the crucial ones enabling you to reach your finishing line.

If we can carry on the metaphor and see our weight loss journey as the race in the story - well – that's a race I have been losing for a long time! As you are reading this book, I am going to assume that your pathway has been like mine: a long and irritatingly unsuccessful journey to lose weight and keep it off. After years of on and off dieting, taking off a few kilos here and putting them back on there, often with a few extra added, I always ended up heavier than when I started out. In fact, I wondered whether dieting itself was a contributing factor in the issues that I was having with weight! Even more reason to stop going down that path and find out what works.

The question is – are you more like the hare or more like the tortoise? I am sure that many of you can identify with the hare-like enthusiasm we have at the start of going on a diet. Oh yes, we say to ourselves – I'm going to stick with this and lose 4 kilos a month, which means I will have reached my goal weight in three months. Or you have a big event coming up in a month and want to lose a certain (usually unrealistic) amount by that date. For some, every Monday is that special day and for many, it is the start of the New Year. But the event comes and goes, Monday comes and turns into Tuesday, and the New Year is barely out of nappies before we have given up and filling the newly created hole with treats.

So, what is it we can learn from this simple and ancient story that will enable us to become more effective in reaching our goals? To answer that question for me, I took a good hard look back at my own life to see if I could identify any patterns of behaviour that kept leading me down the wrong path. Were there connections between my weight journey and anything else going on in my life at the time? Were there times when my life was more like the hare and not enough like the tortoise? Which one was operating when I was successful, and which one wasn't? Here is my story. I invite you to write your own story in your journal and review it to see if you can identify some of your own patterns.

My Story – lessons from losing

I know my diet behaviour didn't really start until I had left home and gone to university, which is when a lot of young people put on a few kilos. Prior to that, I was a skinny little farm girl. We had a typical rural New Zealand upbringing on a small dairy farm. My brothers and sisters and I were all expected to work and take part in the jobs to be done including milking the cows.

We ate simply and always ate together at the table. We ate meat that had been raised on the farm, grass fed of course, potatoes, vegetables, puddings, bottled fruit and cream, always cream, toast with lashings of butter and homemade jam or vegemite and home baking to fill in the gaps. Roasts, casseroles, chicken sometimes for Sunday lunch as the treat it was before chicken was commercialised like it is today. Chances are we helped Grandma catch and despatch said chook beforehand and watched as she stuffed and trussed it up to feed us all.

We were always hungry when we got home from school, so there was a lot of tin-rattling going on to see whether mum had filled them up with louise cake, yoyos or chocolate slice while we were away. A lot of the processed food available now wasn't yet invented, so that wasn't even an issue, although we did sometimes look longingly at those town kids who had shop-bought biscuits for play lunch.

There was some talk at school of diets and some girls went on them or were put on them by their mothers. However, it wasn't an issue for me. I remember having a competition with another girl to see who had the skinniest legs – and it wasn't a good thing. I didn't want to have the skinniest legs!

It wasn't until I left school and went off to university in another town that I felt I had put on some weight. I had been protected from the sort of media that promoted celebrity skinniness but going out into the big wide world and now comparing myself with others opened up a whole new world and I was learning what was expected of me by society at large. Of course, looking back now, I can see that I was nowhere near overweight. I was just a growing young woman with curves in the right places and although more rounded than the skinny child I had been, everything was normal.

However, I obviously bought into the current skinny image of the time, and I ate the occasional desultory meal of a chicken drumstick with a bit of salad (which I thought of as diet food) but as I had to excuse myself from the dinner table and separate myself from the rest of the family that wasn't really destined to work out. By the time I had finished university I certainly wasn't fat or overweight at all –but I felt the beginnings of the struggle to look like the magazines I was looking at said I should. The way I thought about how I looked was changing.

I got married soon after graduating and was a very petite bride. I began a career I loved, but motherhood and domesticity were also calling and I had my first baby in my early twenties. As often happens, we naturally put on weight during that period of our life and I found it difficult to get rid of. I had another child two years later and enjoyed being at home caring for them and running a household. I baked and cooked and sometimes ate too much of my own baking and cooking and got a bit out of balance with everything. I loved it, but I also missed the mind-food that work had given me until then, and dealing with the challenges of raising young children meant I filled in down-time by eating.

The first time I went to a weight loss group, they sensibly wouldn't let me join as I hadn't reached their threshold of what was considered overweight. However, after a bit of effort on my part, I put enough weight on to qualify and so began my typical on again off again relationship with diets.

Over those years I read many diet books, followed the "miracle" diets in the magazines. I invariably got so far into the diet and then bumped up against an obstacle of some sort and came to a halt. The weight went back on with a bit more added besides. Like the hare, I would start off a new diet with a hiss and a roar full of enthusiasm and good intentions. I would typically do well for the first couple of weeks fired up on my enthusiasm and then get ahead of myself - congratulating myself before I had achieved the result. After a while that enthusiasm waned and then eventually bumped up against the reality of life.

Obstacles would suddenly appear. It might be the separate shopping for your diet becomes too difficult for a busy mother, too many family celebrations or work functions, you get sick, break your leg or pull a muscle from overexerting yourself exercising. It always seemed, for example, that whenever I started a new health regime, I would always get sick about two weeks in and that would be the end of that.

Meanwhile, things weren't always so happy at home and as a result, I was eating more than was necessary: something I would identify later as emotional eating. I couldn't really identify what was wrong, but it was uncomfortable and eating seemed to be a way of bringing short-term relief. Not that I realised that was what I was doing. I was experiencing a certain amount of emotional discomfort and, as is often the case, I fed that pain with food. After all, we had all grown up to learn that if we fell over, skinned our knees, and cried loud enough, someone would soon give us an ice-cream or a treat that took our mind off the pain and shut us up. It might take the mind off the pain, but it can sometimes also send the message that, if it hurts, fix it with some immediate gratification, preferably a sweet treat.

What fixed that for me was when I found out why I was not happy and that lead to what some of us recognize as the Divorce Diet. This was the most quick and effective one ever. If you have ever experienced the sort of emotional trauma and stress that can attend the end of a marriage or relationship, you might know what I am talking about. I am not sure whether I ate at all for a month I was so stressed and unhappy. Of course, I ended up losing a lot of weight quickly and although my figure was back to where I really wanted it, I wouldn't recommend getting there in the way I did!

Life carried on and eventually I met another lovely man, re-married and started life with him. Life continued its up and down path, as did my weight, always eventually ending up a little heavier than before. My husband had always worked in a physical occupation and had a naturally lean body type. He also often did a lot of the cooking as I was working outside the home so would serve me up man-size meals which I ate. I've since heard someone referring to this as eating "guy food". Since men have a different metabolism to women with more muscle mass to burn energy, he wasn't affected but I was certainly beginning to be. What was I thinking?

The children were all away from home by this time, so we were a cosy couple. But even though my extra layers didn't bother him so much, it was bothering me. I wanted to fit my clothes and look nice in them. He might have had a lean body type, but I did not! Being on the shorter side and having a fuller figure, extra weight was becoming harder to disguise and more noticeable. It was running out of places to go and starting to go sideways. I was pretty good at dressing for my shape, but I ended up in a particular work role where my job sometimes called for the wearing of Victorian costume with an old-fashioned apron tied around my waist. I did actually have a waist, but it was getting crowded out by my hips and boobs and starting to merge into one. They should have called me Mrs Tiggywinkle – or Mrs Patmore. Not a flattering look.

So yes - I still wanted to look as good as I could with what I had, but I felt it was getting harder and harder to do that as my clothes no longer seemed to fit. It sounds funny, but it's not really when you are staring in your wardrobe wailing that you have nothing to wear. Your bewildered husband is pointing out all the clothes stuffed in there but you know that only about three of them fit.

Then it became a health issue. A blood test showed a cholesterol level that was on the wrong side of where it should be. I noticed aches and pains and had digestive issues. And to top it all off, I experienced a bout of gout. I could not believe it. I was far too young to be experiencing aches and pains, let alone gout! But the blood tests showed that yes, it was exactly that.

As my 50th birthday approached I understandably wanted to lose the kilos I had put on over the past few years so I could look my best. The birthday came and went but my weight did not. Reading back over my journals from the past, I could see that no matter how many times I had started on that journey and set my goals, I still couldn't lose the weight, let alone maintain what I had lost. I didn't want to keep up the trend of putting it on with all the associated health issues – plus I wanted to enter my more mature years looking the best I could and being as healthy as I could.

By this time, I had tried many diets but just could not stick to them. You've heard the old joke about how some people just need to think about going on a diet and they put on weight. It's not a joke. It was happening to me. I could think about it, maybe prepare myself to give it a go, but before I knew it, I would be hunting around looking for something to eat that I knew I didn't really want or need but felt compelled to eat. There was clearly some kind of disordered thinking pattern that had long ingrained itself into my life and I really didn't want to keep going there.

Obviously, what I had tried in the past had not worked in the long term, so what was I going to do differently this time to be successful? As I look back on this story, I can see the connections between what I was thinking, what I was feeling and what was happening with my body. I could even map on a graph where those intersections were.

Lessons from success

When I think back and consider the times when I lost weight or maintained the weight I wanted, I ask myself, what was it about that behaviour that made it effective? And if it was effective then, what about it worked and how can I apply it to my life now?

One of the earliest times I remember when I achieved a good result was when I was a student and had a job over the three months of summer break. I had come home from university where I had put on the customary extra kilos that so often happens when we move away from home and out into the big wide world. To get to my job in the city, I had to get up early to catch the bus, so I grabbed a piece of toast and a cup of tea for breakfast. I wouldn't eat again until lunchtime and ate my homemade sandwich outside in the park. Back on the bus, home at 6.30 ready to sit down with the family to a normal meal eaten together around the table. Nothing had changed in that department, so again, it was usually meat, potatoes, vegetables followed by pudding (with cream, of course).

After those three months, without thinking about it and without trying, I lost weight. I had not intended to, had not really paid much attention, but the routine of eating normal nutritious food, the same dinner as everyone else, keeping myself busy and engaged with life meant that it had happened virtually automatically. Hmmm – food for thought.

We can learn from the success of others as well. Many years later, I worked with a woman who was quite overweight. Let's call her Samantha. I was on another hare-like excursion of going on a diet, so I invited her to come to my weight loss group with me and she declined.

Exhibiting my usual hare-like behaviour, I attended for the first few weeks, lost 3-4 kilos, then something happened that interrupted my concentration. I can't remember what it was, but you and I both know that it is common to bump up against obstacles when we make big changes. As a result, I didn't keep it up. I felt so depressed about the fact that the scales started going in the wrong direction, that I bought chocolate and ice-cream to make me feel better and quietly ended up putting it all back on.

Meanwhile, Samantha decides she is going to get back into shape. And do you know what she did? Every day at lunchtime, she ate the same thing. Every day. She followed a similar pattern for her other meals and shrunk before my eyes. There was no fussing around with different recipes or new kinds of food. Repetition became her friend and accompanied her all the way to the finish line. She behaved like the tortoise and lost weight, and I behaved like a hare and lost it, then gained it plus a bit more. Sound familiar?

Could it be that Samantha was successful because she realised that we sometimes get too complicated trying to fit in with a diet plan we have been given which includes a lot of things we don't normally eat? This has a couple of outcomes that can counteract sustainable weight loss. One is that our busy lives become more complicated when we do the family shopping and must hunt around looking for things on our list we are not familiar with and don't even really like. And aren't our lives complicated enough already?

The other is we spend too much time fussing over recipes and finally we give up and revert to tried and true. It's fairly typical behaviour to get very enthusiastic at the beginning of a new diet but making too many changes too quickly – even if they are good ones – overwhelms us and triggers off the sabotaging of our own good behaviour. This seemed strange, and I wanted to know if there was a reason for it.

Perhaps it was time to learn how to be more like the Tortoise and less like the Hare– take it a bit more slowly, take the time to find out what worked for me at my current stage of life, what I could do to overcome the obstacles that had been stopping me to this point and finally reach my goal. But what were those obstacles? Why had diets not worked for me? What was really going on?

Success Work: Using your journal or workbook write your own life story. Can you identify with my story? What would you say have been the obstacles that stop you when you attempt to diet? If you did lose weight and kept it off in the past, can you remember what sort of behaviour you led to that? What do you think made it effective?

Chapter 2

Stop Starting and Start Stopping

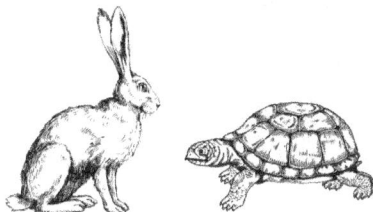

After thinking about my story and the experience of others, I was starting to pick up on some patterns and what some of the problems could be. I was even considering that a big part of the problem lay in the behaviour that traditional diets create in us and that my ongoing failure was not necessarily because I was a 'hopeless lazy, greedy human being with no willpower' or any other of the insults we level at ourselves over the years.

Why dieting has failed

The whole traditional diet process is problematic from the start. I wasn't even overweight when I started, but obviously felt that I didn't measure up somehow and that I needed to be thinner. In hindsight, I could see that I was measuring myself up against what the magazines and TV shows said I should be and look like, that were no less realistic than they are now. They imply there's something wrong with us if we don't look like Kim Kardashian, for example. I'm sure she's a lovely person, but even she doesn't look like Kim Kardashian when she gets up in the morning.

I was buying into the so-called miracle diets of the day that bore no resemblance to my real-life situation and were therefore unsustainable. So as soon as I finished the two weeks (or more like two days) or whatever length of time it was supposed to be and went back to my normal eating pattern, I put anything I may have lost straight back on.

As I found out later, restricting and depriving myself for that short period triggered behaviour that meant my body, unbeknownst to me, interpreted as a sign of impending famine and very sensibly signalled to my appetite to eat even more to put on some extra fat in case famine was threatened again. And losing weight so fast and not eating enough of the right foods meant that most of what I lost was muscle mass anyway. As I also found out later, our bodies burn more energy (calories) to maintain muscle mass. We need every bit of lean muscle tissue we have to facilitate fat burning. Fast, unsafe dieting meant I was losing the very thing I needed the most to burn calories. So not only was I messing with my head and developing disordered thinking, but I was messing with my body and actually ending up in a place opposite to where I wanted to go.

But of course, it wasn't long before I was back trying the next new one because now I really needed to lose some weight! It's no wonder a massive weight loss industry has been created in the last few decades. What a business opportunity. Create a problem by telling everyone they are not acceptable as they are and need to be thinner. Create fear of being fat. Then offer the solution – their diet – which might work if you stick to it. But we already know that is impossible because clearly none of us can stick to it.

Everyone knows that if you just eat salad and poached fish or chicken all the time then you will be skinny. But because that is not sustainable, we give up. We feel like failures and therefore indulge in the opposite behaviour. We put weight back on and so the cycle begins. You won't have to wait long for the next new miracle cure because come summer there will be one in every magazine you buy or showing up in your social media feed and you, ever hopeful, will jump on the bandwagon and give it another go.

Now, not only are you fatter, but you feel guilty for failing and you feel even worse about yourself. So, you add disordered thinking to your list of what is making you fat. We use food for a lot of reasons that it was never designed for – in particular, hoping that it will take us out of a negative state and back to being happy. Emotional eating, boredom eating, procrastination eating, punish yourself eating and just plain old overeating even though you know you are not hungry eating. Eating and food ends up having very little to do with nutrition or fellowship – the very thing it is designed for.

We may gain knowledge along the way and, in fact, some of you are diet experts specialising in calorie counting. Who can list all the diets they have done over the years? Who knows the calorific content of a chocolate bar at thirty paces? We are all unique beings living in a challenging world, so even if we have the knowledge, how do we apply it in a life full of real interruptions and the other obstacles life brings us? Has that knowledge set you free? Has it been the right knowledge that applies to your own life?

Traditional diets assume that life is a continuous uninterrupted journey, whereas it's very clear that life is not like that. There are hard times, boring times, exciting times, happy times, and everything in between. Unexpected changes happen unexpectedly. Life is full of ups and downs. Traditional diets are not tailored to match where we are in life. They certainly don't allow for the family celebrations that are part of life. If you're not allowed to eat cake, what happens on your birthday?

We are all different, so a one size fits all diet will never fit all. Our bodies change over time as we produce children, get older, get slower, or whatever the case may be for you. What you need to eat as a lactating mother is going to differ from the nutritional requirements of a menopausal woman. The needs of a young athletic sportswoman or man are going to be very different to someone the same age whose main sport is sitting on the couch gaming and eating a diet consisting mainly of highly processed fast food. There is a natural ebb and flow to our days, months, and years. There are seasons in life just as there are seasons in the natural world. Most traditional diets don't allow for any of that.

A lot of the diets I went on were simply unrealistic. They specified foods I'd never heard of, foods out of season, foods simply not available, or that no one else in the household was going to eat. Shopping for weird foods and preparing separate meals just added another level of complexity to an already busy life. They were just too far removed from normal life and actually, as we are going to find out, our brains love normal – even if it's bad for us.

Most diets focus on the calorie content of food so we develop the mindset of seeing food only as calories or fuel and therefore give no thought to the quality of food we put into our bodies. Imagine if we did that to our cars? Hands up those of you who, while following a traditional diet of 1500 calories a day, worked out that if all calories are equal, and a chocolate bar was 500 calories, you chose it over a big chicken salad sandwich?

Eventually, when we are well and truly caught up in the struggle, they keep lying to us and saying we can lose a lot of weight quickly if only we try hard enough. It is a powerful message, and I kept getting sucked into it. But if I've spent many years putting on weight and given no thought as to why or what sort of environment I had created to support being at that weight – what's going to happen when I don't lose the weight in that magically short period of time? My unrealistic expectations were going to cause me to be discouraged and give up again.

Losing weight slowly was never an option because who wanted to do that? Our world is set up for instant results, instant gratification. Think about all the transformation shows in the media these days – your body, your house, your garden. The diet industry knows that and taps straight into that vein. In fact, when I was telling someone about the message behind this book of losing weight slowly over time, she said to me that no one was ever going to buy it. There's a classic marketing strategy about selling what people want (or think they want) but giving them what they need. This book is about giving you what you need because what you want (the miracle fast permanent weight loss diet) hasn't worked so far.

But most of all, I realised that diets hadn't worked because they never really addressed the reasons we were fat in the first place. They had exacerbated the problem by creating disordered thinking and behaviour that made us put on even more weight – but never answered the question about why we do what we do even though we know better. And those reasons are not usually visible ones.

Unfortunately, the symptoms of those invisible reasons are clearly visible as they hang out on our hips and thighs and arms and boobs, and everywhere else excess weight goes. By the time you have been a failed dieter for more than a few years, you have to consider the possibility that it's the inward condition that is causing the outer manifestation. Is it possible that our bodies are desperately trying to signal to us that something is wrong, and you need to make some changes? That does not come into the traditional diet equation at all. Putting some time and effort into uncovering the reasons you are overweight in the first place and what has stopped you in the past will be crucial to finally winning this race.

Dieting behaviour is a big contributor to the problem of being overweight, but there are others. When I was growing up, there was little in the way of processed or altered foods available as options. When my kids were growing up, that was starting to be an issue and now we have an entire generation who have been raised on diets of highly processed so-called foods that bear little resemblance to what food is really meant to be. The effect on our bodies has been to basically blow out our whole biochemical systems and we've all gone into inflammation overdrive.

Our bodies don't recognise the laboratory altered fats that are presented to us in trans-fats, nor were they designed to recognise the altered sugars delivered in the highly processed carbohydrates of the fast food era. Our tastebuds have been almost cauterized by those super highly flavoured but very tasty foods so that when we want to eat in a more wholesome way, the foods that we should eat seem to be flavourless in comparison.

Our livers, kidneys and other digestive organs are overloaded by not only the food but all the other chemicals in our environment so can't function as well as they should. Did you know that the liver is one of our best allies in getting rid of excess fat from our bodies? We do not do it any favours with the modern way of eating or living. I was talking to a girl at the check-out of our local grocery store who even though she was still at secondary school and aged sixteen, had been diagnosed with fatty liver disease, something that used to be alcohol related but is now showing up in younger and younger people who don't even drink alcohol.

The same generation who have had their bodies overwhelmed by fast foods have also grown up with a massive media onslaught from the minute they are placed in front of the telly with messages to eat whatever fast food is currently being pushed. It's no wonder there's such a problem. On the one hand, we are bombarded with messages to eat this or drink that, and on the other we're told we must look like the super skinny fit-looking image that is just as prevalent in the media. Is it any wonder there is so much confusion and anxiety out there? We are suffering the consequences in the obesity statistics, incidences of metabolic illnesses and so on in increasingly younger people, cardiovascular issues, and all kinds of illnesses. The playing field is really stacked against us.

Lifestyle factors such as the all-pervading stress and anxiety that most of us live with in the modern world can play havoc with our hormones and prevent us from losing fat. Lack of or poor sleep has been shown to be a factor, as is lack of exercise as part of daily life. Even our gut health can be part of the equation.

And then there are the underlying medical conditions you may have, sometimes as the consequences of the above type of eating, that you may not even know about yet. The obvious ones are metabolic like diabetes or gout, various forms of cancer, thyroid problems, autoimmune conditions. If there is ever a time to eat right for our bodies and getting rid of excess weight, it is now. Old age is not for the faint-hearted and neither is it for the fat or unfit.

It's not a pretty picture out there of either the way the traditional diets set us up for failure, or the way our whole environment seems to be programmed to support being sick and overweight. Please don't get all depressed and give up yet, however. There are the seeds of solution in my story as well! I had some successes and learned from the success of others but it was once I turned my attention to my behaviour around the problem of being overweight that I started to make some inroads towards those solutions.

Which brings us back to the fable. What profound truth was lurking there under cover of what is commonly thought of as a children's story? Which approach was I operating in when I was engaging in unsuccessful results and what could I identify in the behaviour when I was successful? Was I behaving more like the hare or more like the tortoise?

It brought me to the first guidepost you will find on this journey – and that is – to stop the dieting behaviour altogether. Guidepost One is to stop dieting.

Success Work: I've outlined some of the problems with traditional diets and how they have contributed to our failure. Which ones apply to you? What other reasons can you give? Make a list of the reasons why you personally think you have become overweight.

Stage 2

Getting A New Strategy

If I want to win the race I need a new strategy. My old one doesn't work.

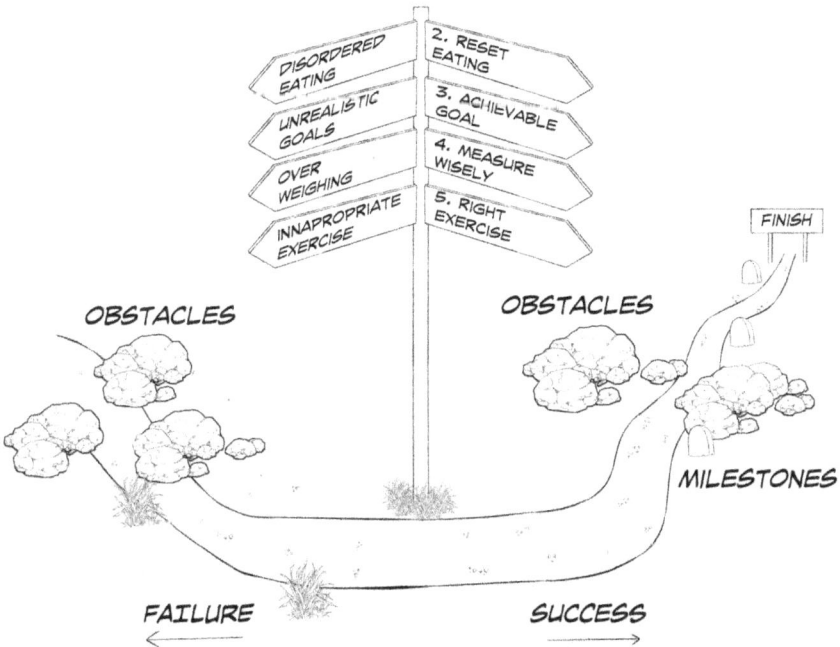

DISORDERED EATING

UNREALISTIC GOALS

OVER WEIGHING

INNAPROPRIATE EXERCISE

2. RESET EATING

3. ACHIEVABLE GOAL

4. MEASURE WISELY

5. RIGHT EXERCISE

FINISH

OBSTACLES

OBSTACLES

MILESTONES

FAILURE

SUCCESS

Chapter 3

The Hare Diet

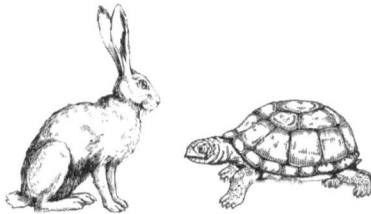

What does it mean to act less like a hare and more like a tortoise? What does this lovely old fable mean and why is it so inherently useful for our success? Well, let us take a quick look at the behaviour of each and see how effective it was.

Let's start with the hare. It is only natural to start with her (yes-she is a girl!) as she is naturally the one that you would notice first if she walked into a room. Full of energy and talk and probably the life of the party. I love hares. I love seeing them loping around the paddocks near where I live and boy - can they run! It would have been such a joke to imagine the hare and the tortoise racing. In fact, it would seem an impossible contest. So, what did the hare do in this story that prevented her from winning the race?

- Like us at the beginning of a new diet, she started off with loads of enthusiasm and confidence but ran out of steam not too far into the race.
- She was all about the starting line and not enough about the finishing line.
- Maybe she thought the finishing line would always be there and was hers by right?
- She certainly got easily side-tracked and lost focus on the job at hand.
- She took a very short-term approach to the task at hand and went after her immediate desires by eating those cabbages and taking that nap in the middle of the race rather than delay until the job had been done.
- She certainly didn't take advantage of her strengths and didn't do the work necessary to reach the goal even though she had the natural ability.
- She was a little overconfident in her ability but couldn't come up with the goods – all talk and no results.

Those are some I can think of – and they all seemed strangely familiar to me. Ponder on the hare yourself and see where you can identify your own behaviours.

You have already seen in my story and can probably identify in your own, the way we typically approach going on a diet. In fact, the approach of the hare has come to mean in our culture an approach that is fast and furious with little to sustain it in the long term. I will not bore you with stories about every time I started at the gym or on a diet because you are probably already well acquainted with that story in your own life. Suffice to say, I would often begin a diet with high hopes, lots of confidence and maybe a lot of talk about how I was going to do this and that only to crash and burn within a couple of weeks (or days) into my journey.

Sure, that feeling of possibility and excitement to start with was great and pleasurable, but it was never actually enough to carry me to the end of the race. People are great at starting things but not so good at finishing. I would like to finish things now thanks very much. Time to reach goals, especially now that I am old enough to know what those goals are. Time to put into practice the behaviour of the tortoise, who did actually finish the race.

Now, consider the behaviour of the tortoise in our fable.

- She (also a girl!) started off quietly and with little fanfare, even though the goal seemed very far away and the other contender was far better equipped to reach it.
- She put one foot in front of the other and kept going and going until she had reached the finish line.
- Even though the goal seemed out of reach, she broke it down into achievable steps and consistently followed through on those steps.
- She did what came naturally. She didn't do something too far outside the normalcy zone. Maybe if she was more like the hare, she could have decided to dance or maybe skip her way to the goal and therefore potentially reach it earlier.
- The tortoise did what she knew worked for her and repeated it at regular intervals, and naturally reached the finish line.
- She didn't waste time and energy or give up by thinking of all the reasons she couldn't possibly win, especially against such an obviously talented foe.

- She didn't make excuses about not having the right gear or not having the time.
- She just got on with the job.
- Maybe most important of all – she *stayed in the race.*

Not as exciting and glamourous as the hare – but clearly as a strategy, it was way more effective. Perhaps having the right strategy is an important part of success? If you think of our struggle to lose weight as being a race or a journey, then consider how someone who is successful at winning may approach it.

An elite athlete who is in the game to win will have a coach who can identify the strengths and weaknesses that the athlete has with a view to correcting the weaknesses and maximising the strengths. If we are going to win at this race, then we need a gameplan that works. Having the right approach is the beginning of having the right strategy. Slowing right down to the pace of the tortoise; taking the time to understand what the right steps are; what the right goal is; identifying and overcoming weaknesses; learning the tools that will equip you for success; and getting your environment organised to support your success, are all part of the approach of the *Tortoise Diet Method.*

I finally realised that I had been on the hare diet for most of my life and it was getting me nowhere I wanted to go. Perhaps it was time to consider this new method instead.

The Tortoise Diet Method

Considering the lessons learned and observations made in my own life and those of others around me, especially concerning the way traditional dieting had not worked and had possibly been a major contributor to weight gain, I thought about 'what if'.

What if I had never started on a diet in the first place but continued eating the way I had in a normal regular fashion, adjusting naturally to where I was in whatever stage of life, listening to my body when it said *that's enough* or *I feel bad when I eat that so don't eat it?*

What if I had continued that path? Would I have gained this distorted and dangerous relationship that I now had with food? Would I have a weight problem?

What if, instead of the usual three times each year where I determine to lose weight, lose a few kilos, and then a few weeks later put back on what I lost with extra besides – what if I did something different?

What did the tortoise do when venturing on that journey one step at a time but break down the big goal of the race into many small steps. So, what if I broke down my weight loss journey into really, *really* manageable steps?

In fact, what if I lower my expectations and increase the time over which to achieve that goal?

What if I aim to lose, and keep off – wait for it - *1 kilo per month?* And what If I made the length of the race – wait for it - *one entire year?*
And what if I did not put myself on a diet, but just *ate three normal nutritious meals a day?*
And what if I stopped weighing myself obsessively all the time *but only weighed myself once a month, if at all?*

Keep reading! I can hear you all groaning from here. 1 kilo a month! What is that all about? But bear with me. What if you make a couple of small but significant changes to your eating that won't take it too far from what is normal for you to start with, doesn't require disruption to the rest of your household, that doesn't require lots of fussing around with unfamiliar foods and scales but meant you lost at least 1 kilo per month? Wouldn't that be a lot better than what you have done in the past?

Metric Conversion.
1 Kg = 2.2 pounds.
12 Kg = 26.45 pounds

If you lost 1 kilo a month without thinking too much about it, by the end of the year you would have lost 12 kilos. Isn't that a lot better than taking off and putting back on some unrealistic amount? You would have done it slowly and consistently, learning along the way, giving your body time to adjust to the small changes, your mind to embed the new habits that are the key to the *Tortoise Diet Method*, and therefore more likely to keep it off.

And during that period, you are going to discover how to make those changes sustainable. You actively seek what has been stopping you and getting to the bottom of self-sabotaging behaviour, then not only will you have lost some weight but you will have developed the right mindset and habits that will become the tools you need for keeping the weight off.

If you have just read this and cried out to yourself - "but I need to lose XXX (insert your number in here) kilos/pounds!" think about the hare and the tortoise. You can theoretically lose 3-4 kilos (6-8lbs) a month safely and consequently lose nearly 45 kilos (100lbs) a year if you could stick to a diet for that period of time.

The trap for many of us is that like the hare we start out with lots of enthusiasm at the beginning trying to lose an unrealistic amount in an unrealistic timeframe. We falter at the first hurdle, give up and put more weight back on so that by the end of the year not only have you not lost what you wanted but you have gained more. The next year you have more to lose than the year before.

Keep doing that year after year and the trend is not pretty. Look at your weight-loss history to date. Where is that trend line going? It may go up and down (or more like down and then up) each time you embark on another traditional diet, but you may well be ending up a little heavier each time. The trend line is heading in the general direction of north. It does not take much to figure out that the health issues tied in with being overweight and unhealthy –let alone fitting into your clothes – could potentially become quite problematic over time if you do nothing to correct the curve.

Compare that with the tortoise and slowly but steadily aim for a reasonable and achievable monthly goal and you are much more likely to reach it. If you still have more to lose, then follow the same principles the following year. You are far more likely to reach your goals over the same period doing it this way than the more common stop / start dieting we tend to do. Most of us would be happy to lose 10-12 kilos (22-26lbs) and keep it off. If we have more to lose, keep going armed with your new insights and knowledge, get on with living life and take the focus off the thought of dieting. By following this method, the tendency to put on weight as we get older is reversed and, as a result, we are healthier and more gorgeous as we get older.

What a revelation! And it's achievable. *Everyone can lose 1 kilo per month - including you!*

So how does this all work? How can I incorporate the lessons of the tortoise and the hare and apply them to my own life? Here are the three main principles that make up your new strategy for success. I'm going to call them the Guideposts. You are in the race to the finish line so you will need these guideposts to show you the way. The first guidepost has already been covered in chapter 2 and that is to stop dieting behaviour altogether. These next three may seem oddly mundane and not what you were expecting, but sometimes the best and most effective ideas are the simplest.

PRINCIPLES OF THE TORTOISE DIET STRATEGY

Guidepost 2. Reset your eating

Eat three normal nutritious moderate meals a day, not too different from your current normal, making sure that those meals provide you with the nutrition you need. Eat enough to feel satisfied and keep you going until the next meal. If you cannot make it from lunch to dinner without getting over hungry, then include a nutritious mid-afternoon snack. Reduce treat food to the occasional and enjoy it with others as part of life's celebrations.

Guidepost 3. Achievable Goal

Aim to lose 1 kilo per month over the course of the year. Like the tortoise, break down the journey into small increments of time with a realistic goal of 1 kilo (2.2lbs) a month. The small daily changes you make will take you steadily towards your achievable goal. Don't try to do it by last week but extend the time over a year to give yourself time to deal with your particular obstacles and acquire the knowledge needed to take the right steps.

Guidepost 4. Measure Wisely

Weigh yourself once a month. Whatever that figure is, even though it might be more than 1 kilo, it becomes your new starting point for the following month. Your next goal is to lose 1 kilo in the new month starting from whatever that new figure is.

Getting Started

The great thing about the Tortoise Diet is that it doesn't require money, special equipment or weird foods. You can start right now, using what you have and if you do what you can – you will get there in the end. This is why I have put the chapter on the key principles of the diet early in the book – you can get started right away. You don't need to wait around until the conditions are right. You will learn that to be sustainable, your diet has to fit in with your life or it won't work, so, you might as well start now.

A set of good scales would be useful. In the remote possibility that you don't have a set of scales at your house (you may have thrown them out already) and don't want to buy any, then use an item of clothing as a reference point. A piece of clothing that you love and used to fit, for example. Try them on and see how far apart the button is. I'm thinking of a pair of jeans, for example. Take a picture for reference. You will discover that weight loss itself is not necessarily a true reflection of fat loss, so take your key measurements and note them down in your journal with the current date as another indicator.

Most of us have enough everyday food in the cupboard or the fridge to eat normally. We will go more into understanding what to eat later on, but in the meantime, make sure you include some good protein, increase the vegetable or salad portion, and reduce your starchy carbohydrate portion of the meal. Cut out processed foods as much as you can.

Start with what you know now and make just enough of a change to begin moving in the right direction without rocking the boat too much. Then, as you learn what works most effectively for you at your stage of life, you can start to gradually change toward the direction that gives you the results you are looking for. But you don't jump to that space in your first few weeks. It can be too much of a shock to the system and you won't be able to sustain it. If you make changes too fast it will only be a matter of time before the old reasons you failed in the past show up to stop you all over again and that's what we want to avoid.

Chapter 4

The Great Reset

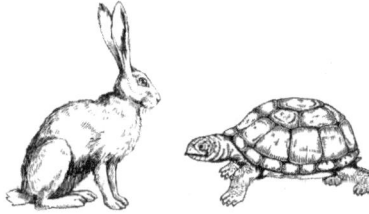

Eat three normal nutritious meals a day

Wow. Eat three normal meals a day. It is crazy that this has become such a loaded statement. In a world overwhelmed with conflicting food messages and cooking programmes everywhere you look, it is easy to drown out the memory of what is normal and nutritious for us to eat. Eating normally as in the old fashioned three regular nutritious satisfying and enjoyable meals a day without too much in between is hardly a radical notion, but not one normally associated with weight loss.

One problem with that statement is that some of us no longer remember what is normal and some have never known what is normal. Some more traditional cultures would look at you like you were crazy if you asked them what normal food was. Normal food is food you grew up with that comes from your region, made with recipes used by your family, your village and community and therefore rooted in your culture. They would be ones that you would regularly serve to your family.

Even in New Zealand before the 1980s - before the time when processed and fast foods became easy or convenient choices -we had our own traditional nutritious food as part of our normal. Protein, usually grass-fed meat, fish, milk, cheese, carbohydrates in the form of potatoes, good bread, loads of home-grown vegetables, plus the occasional treat of home baking made with real flour, real sugar and real butter not including artificial colours, flavours or altered fats and sugars. That was normal then, and it's still a very good normal to have now. In fact, I would go so far to say that it's highly likely if we had just kept eating that way and not got ourselves all messed up with food fads and restrictive diet type behaviour, we would not have the weight problems we do now.

Think about it. If you had just carried on eating normally and moderately and not messed up your relationship with food, over-using it for all sorts of reasons quite unrelated to nutrition, then you probably would not be in this position now.

Remember how I told you about how I "accidentally" lost weight by eating my usual three meals and nothing else? I didn't do anything special outside of eating normal meals at normal mealtimes. What I learned from my own experiences in going on diets over the years is that once you restrict yourself at mealtimes, you become more vulnerable to the trap that high calorie snacks eaten between meals often provide and here's the problem with that. It is the snacks we eat outside of those three normal meals a day that can be the major contributor to weight gain.

Is it not true that what we eat most of outside of normal mealtimes, at morning tea, afternoon tea or after dinner is cake, biscuits, lollies, chips, and chocolate? That, my friends, is where the sneaky unneeded calories lurk. The pleasure-giving qualities last only as long as the time you are eating them and once down the hatch, as the old saying goes, are pretty hard to dispatch.

So why start with what is normal for you? One of the biggest problems with sustaining a new diet is that it can mean eating unfamiliar foods that are too far outside our normalcy zone and this has contributed to our failure to stick with them. Traditional diets often suck us in by promising quick results if we make all these changes all at once. The problem with that is our bodies don't like unfamiliar, they don't like change and will put up the sort of resistance we recognize as those obstacles that stop us dieting. If you've ever been in a beautiful big boat sailing out there on the ocean you will know that you can't suddenly stop and change direction without creating some kind of massive turbulence. The same goes for us. This is more an evolution rather than revolution kind of a method so slow down, then stop the old behaviour first before slowly implementing the new effective ones.

We all have developed our own special comfort zone of eating that may be normal for you but is not actually working. It's possibly even causing you to become unwell and probably overweight. So even though you may be apparently wanting to take good positive steps in your life towards making those good food choices (and good life choices!) this old hidden but powerful part of you interprets that as unfamiliar and therefore dangerous. It sets about sabotaging that new behaviour so you can go right back to being good old familiar you.

We already know that the more you step outside your comfort zone and make lots of changes all at once, you are going to run into some kind of obstacle that will stop you. Of course, the more changes you make, the better the results will be that you will get – but if you could do that already, then you probably wouldn't be reading this book. The *Tortoise Diet Method* will require a little extra of you, but not too much too soon. Push gently against the boundaries of your comfort zone and extend them gradually over time to cheat the pushback.

The slow and steady approach of the *Tortoise Diet Method* aims to sneak in under the radar and evade this normalcy bias by making sure those meals are not too different from your current normal to start with, but it is important that those meals provide you with the nutrition you need and there is enough to be satisfied and keep you going until the next meal.

What you are aiming to do is not so much go on a diet but learn how to eat enough from your regular balanced meals to keep you nourished so you are not looking for snacks in between. It is not so much about restricting any food groups as much as learning that when you eat more of certain foods, you feel much better. Listening to what your body tells you about what you eat will tell you what works for you. Heartburn, indigestion, bloating, and nausea are all indicators that whatever you ate does not agree with you so stop adding it to your diet – or at the very least reduce its use.

And then as you learn what works best for you, that keeps you not just starting to look fantastic but to feel fantastic, you harness the power of this normalcy bias that has been an obstacle in the past and your turn it into one of the most powerful tools for success by making it your new normal! This new normal over time will effectively be keeping you at the right weight without all that old effort. That is what I mean when I say normal.

There are some other great reasons to eat this way. Starting a practice of normal ordered behaviour with regular meals will counteract the disordered thinking you have probably acquired. You know, the one where you say I haven't had any lunch so I'll just eat this cake. Or I haven't eaten all day and I am starving, so I'm going to eat everything in sight whether it serves my goal or not. It is a poor strategy to miss meals and then overeat the next one. But it occurs way too often in those who think they lose weight by eating less. I don't recommend missing meals at all unless you are doing it as part of a deliberate and safe fasting plan, but I suggest you hold that off until you have healed yourself of this disordered thinking.

Nutritious

Nutritious means getting what your body needs to function at an optimum health level, protecting you from disease and making you glow with good health. You get nutrition from eating a wide range of foods that will provide you with what the body needs: macro nutrients such as good quality protein, good quality fats and complex carbohydrates plus the micronutrients of vitamins and minerals vital for the proper functioning of a healthy body. It does not need over processed foods, altered foods that the body does not recognize, or empty calories.

Meeting your nutritional needs is an important part of the *Tortoise Diet Method*. You may not realize it, but many obese people are suffering from malnutrition. If your body is not getting what it needs in terms of nutrition then it will keep signalling it needs more food in a desperate attempt to get the nutrients it requires. This could be one reason behind overeating behaviour. If you keep responding to that hunger signal by continue to supply it with nutritionally challenged junk food, you can end up getting caught in a sad cycle. Combine that with a culture that has become disconnected from its traditional food, and you end up with more and more people losing the health and weight battle.

In the *Tortoise Diet Method*, starting where you are means you start with what is familiar to you but then gradually tweak that over time to include more of the foods that are going to be effective in reaching your end goal. The key here is that you have time to make those new foods so much a part of your life that they become your new familiar and then eventually your new normal. You also give your body time to adjust to a new set point.

So, start there, but as you learn what works for you and suits your lifestyle, make minor adjustments to that meal to bring it into the effective zone. The small changes you can make straight away are to make sure you have some protein at every meal, add something fermented for gut health, add a good serve of vegetables at lunch and dinner and include a couple of pieces of fruit somewhere in that. Then just get on and eat those three normal meals a day, making sure they contain enough of what your body needs to keep it satisfied until the next meal. That way you are not looking for empty calories in between.

Moderate

When I say moderate, I mean to eat enough to satisfy you until the next meal. For some of you, this may mean eating more than you have allowed yourself before and it may take a while to overcome the fear of doing that. I don't mean eating more junk but eating more whole nourishing food. For others, it will mean pulling back on the portions and listening to your body when it tells you it has had enough. That means starting today with cooking the normal sort of meal you have always cooked for your family, then eating enough to satisfy your hunger and not going for seconds.

Eating this way is going to reconnect you to an old friend – one you may not have been aware of for a very long time. If you eat in this moderate way, taking your nutrition at three regular daily meals, then you might have a funny feeling 2-3 hours after your last meal that you can't quite recognize but vaguely recall. That feeling is hunger and if you can reconnect to this feeling, it will not only guide you to timing mealtimes and choosing well, but it will increase your pleasure. Eating something delicious when you are a little bit hungry makes it all the more delicious. Learning to love this feeling rather than fearing it is a good tip for success.

Eating when you are a little bit hungry rather than over hungry also sends the message to your limbic system that there is plenty out there in the world and it doesn't have to go into restrictive mode. On the other hand, having too long a gap between meals can mean you are very hungry and the danger there is overeating the wrong foods. It may take a little while to get that balance right.

Think of the hunger and satisfaction ratio as a spectrum. At one end is "Very hungry- could eat a horse and want one right now," to "post-Christmas dinner I feel so full I can hardly move."

I am going to suggest that both extremes are unpleasant and uncomfortable places to be. Neither is going to put you in a place where you are going to sustain your behaviour.

Somewhere in the middle of that spectrum is where you should aim to be eating. The left-hand end moves from the extreme over hungry, down the scale to the very hungry, then pleasantly hungry. On the other side of the fulcrum is pleasantly satisfied, a bit too full, then uncomfortably full. For the Tortoise Diet, aim to stay in that central zone most of the time and this brings me to the snacks department.

Over hungry	Very hungry	Pleasantly hungry	Meal time	Pleasantly satisfied	A bit too full	Uncomfortably full
Pain	Pain	Pleasure	Pleasure	Pleasure	Pain	Pain

Diagram: The Hunger Scale.

Snacks

It is important for sustainable weight loss that you do not keep grazing or snacking all day long. This interferes with the natural digestion process and can also cause multiple spikes in your blood sugar throughout the day especially if you are snacking on processed or sweet foods. Stopping eating in between meals or after your evening one is one of the most effective habits you can do as we all know it's in those snack foods that the calories live.

There is room, however for a snack in the afternoon. I suggest that staying in that central zone means not going over three hours without eating. So, I have breakfast as late as I can, then lunch 3 -4 hours later, which means that it can be five to six hours until dinner time unless I act like my Grandma, who used to have her evening meal at about 5 o'clock. If your time is your own and it suits you, then do it. But if not, the five to six-hour gap is too much, especially after a hard day at work.

When we are tired and worn out, we are vulnerable to temptation. Any good intentions we had of eating well can disappear out the window. If you have ever heard of the word "Hangry" you will understand that can apply to this time of the day. We are much more likely to forgo good choices and opt for convenience and empty calories over nutrition if we get into that state unless we prepare for it. So yes. Please eat something around 3-4.00 pm or at the time that works best for you. Ideally, make that snack contain some good protein and fat in it to counteract any insulin spikes from your old sugar-based options.

Here are some suggestions:

- A handful of nuts plus a small piece of fruit,
- A boiled egg, or a piece of cheese and some fruit,
- A piece of high fibre toast with peanut butter or avocado,
- Some celery and peanut butter,
- Left over chicken wrapped in lettuce,
- A couple of plain biscuits and a cup of tea.

This should help you to safely get to your evening mealtime. This is also why it is important to plan your meals and make it as easy as possible to sustain this way of eating. You are far more likely to be successful if you have a meal planned and ready to eat when you need it.

A key benefit of this method is that it offers a reset which will help you correct the disordered eating and thinking behaviours picked up from years of dieting. If we make sure our meals cover our nutritional requirements, we reduce the incidence of cravings, feelings of being over-hungry and the danger of choosing the wrong foods. We also eliminate the cycle of eating rubbish, putting on weight, feeling like rubbish, eating more rubbish to cheer yourself up, and so on.

Celebrations

Food in most cultures is not just calories but fellowship and community, so this is where the exceptions to the rule come in. If you are eating well at each regular meal, and eating just enough to get the nutrients you require so you are not starving between meals, then from time to time, enjoy treats such as delicious cake or whatever that might be for you. If there is a birthday or other celebration, then join in and enjoy!

Choose the food rather than let the food choose you. It is easier to do this if you are not overly hungry when you go to an event. This is a management issue and you need to think in terms of risk minimization. Never get so hungry that you overeat the kinds of foods that trigger old behaviour. There is a lot more pleasure in eating less but making sure it is really good quality food, than over-eating a lot of low-quality food or drink. I got to where I would only eat sweet treats if it was something I really felt like or wanted. I would then take the time to really enjoy that treat and absolutely not feel guilty about it.

There is another trick here that some people use called the five-bite trick. Most of the time, it is only in the first five bites that we experience all the things we associate with the big slab of chocolate cake or whatever it is. So really savour those and then stop when it just gets boring. Practice having a bit of what you fancy and enjoying it. That is what skinny chefs do. They taste and that is it.

Same with alcohol. One nice glass of good wine savoured slowly rather than several glasses of marginal forgettable alcohol became my new normal. Eating like this should be part of a normal life, and that is what you are aiming for. What is not normal is starving yourself and then eating five pieces of cake in one sitting.

I developed what I found to be an effective habit of getting into the routine of eating regularly and repeating meals during the week when I was focused on work, and then enjoying eating in a more relaxed way over the weekend. It is not restricting so much as choosing to eat at the lower end of my requirements so that when I eat at the higher end on the weekend, it will all balance out.

This is what we are going for in the *Tortoise Diet Method*. Not just eating normal healthy whole foods, not too far removed from your general diet, but also relegating food to where it belongs, as nutritious and delicious, but not the whole focus of life. Being engaged in living a meaningful life leaves little time for focusing on food and wondering where my next snack was going to come from.

Chapter 5

Wait Not Weight

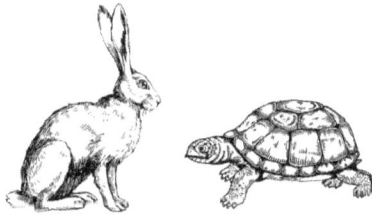

ONE KILOGRAM A MONTH OVER ONE YEAR.

One kilo a month....

know it seems counterintuitive to aim for only 1 kilo a month, especially when the success gurus talk about aiming high and having big goals. That may (but clearly doesn't) work for the hares amongst us, but we know how that has ended in the past. I am not saying that at some point you can't increase that figure, but I suggest you start small, get some really good effective success habits in place first, then build on those.

Yes – I know that the thought of only losing a potential 12 kilos in a year may not sound exciting or inspirational, but if you have never actually achieved it before, then it should be! Lower your expectations a bit and see how that works for you.

What I found inspiring about it was the possibility that I could successfully achieve it rather than repeatedly failing to reach the higher goals I would previously set for myself. Afterall, how has having those big audacious goals worked for you in the past, anyway? How did you even come up with the figure of what you think of as your goal weight? If you are caught up in the social media message of being perfect and being super skinny, then you will continue to set yourself up for failure, especially if you are a menopausal woman for example.

There are tables of weight ranges out there but they are not always useful as they are very generalized and do not take all things into consideration. I had a male friend who was short but very muscley and so showed up technically as obese on the chart yet he clearly wasn't. It might be a silly question to ask, but are you even fat in the first place? Getting a clear and realistic assessment of your actual situation is a useful exercise as well as getting a clear and realistic weight goal.

Starting with a realistic goal is more likely to make it achievable. You are far better off to start with aiming to get your weight to trend down however small that may be to start with and let your weight balance itself out naturally rather than trying to become the weight you were when you were eighteen. It may be possible, but at what cost? The *Tortoise Diet Method* goes for that balance between enjoying life by eating well and living well without the rules and restrictions of a traditional diet.

There is another important reason for the low bar being set here. It will rebuild the pattern of success in your life. You may not realise it, but if you have been a typical yoyo dieter, then your body is probably not going to take you seriously at first. You will need to consistently take those small achievable steps for a bit longer than a couple of weeks in order to correct that pattern.

So how did I come up with this idea of one kilo a month? One thing I noticed when I was doing well on a diet program is that I would strictly follow the plan but sometimes have a bit extra here and there. I could still lose a kilo a week doing that. So, I started thinking, why go through this extra pain of being overly restrictive just to lose weight quickly? Would I be happier and have more success if I spread out the loss over a bit more time and ease up on the restriction? I would still get the same results – it is just they would take a little longer to achieve.

So, what if I reduced my target goal over the time period allocated (1 kilo a month rather that 1 kilo a week) which meant I wasn't so restrictive about limiting my calorie intake as a traditional diet? Surely that would be more sustainable. The payoff for not losing so much is that I could eat more in line with my normal pattern while still being mindful of choosing wisely, and therefore be more likely to stay on the diet.

One kilo is small enough to be sustainable in the real world. By that I mean that life never flows smoothly. We don't always have control over events or what goes on in the lives of our family, so there will be times when even though we might be making good food choices, that life happens. There are always going to be interruptions to our routine; there is a party to go to, we have a bad day and a bit of a blowout. A full and meaningful life will have times of feast and times of famine and always has done. This method allows for normal eating patterns – some days you eat more and sometimes you eat less, depending on what is going on in your life.

You need to factor in the occasional treats as well because we are human and need them. Contrary to popular opinion, we just don't need them every day or at every meal. Life is not a perpetual kid's birthday party and we are no longer children. But yes, we will and should indulge now and then. So, to be sustainable over time, a sensible approach takes that into account.

This also provides a solution to one of the fundamental problems that years of dieting has produced in us and that is the disordered thinking around food many of us have developed. For example, if you eat a big slab of chocolate cake when you are on a traditional type diet, chances are you feel guilty that you have fallen off the wagon and therefore a failure. So, what do you do? Eat the entire cake, of course, often while running a whole stream of self abusive thoughts to go along with that. We tend to catastrophise any slip up and then use it as an excuse to give up and just go the whole hog. Realistically, no-one is going to go through life without having a treat every now and again, so build it in to your way of life. The *Tortoise Diet Method* allows for that so helps to rebuild normal thinking and behaviour around food.

Learn to eat mostly in a way where you eat just enough to be satisfied and meet your nutritional needs, and that will counterbalance the times when you eat more than your body needs, but your soul might enjoy.

You can lose more than just 1 kilo of course and probably will, but we want to take this slow and steady and make it permanent. Don't get overconfident too soon and take on too much change before you have laid your new foundations. Failure is not an option this time. So don't be discouraged about just 1 kilo a month – it is a sensible and achievable goal and will bring you results.

Over a year....

A year may seem like a mighty long time, especially when you think you have a lot to lose. But in giving yourself more time, you are giving yourself a wonderful gift.

Do you feel a massive sense of anxiety when you see the weight going on despite all your efforts to lose it? Do you go down a familiar path of negative self-talk, beating yourself up for failing yet again and getting into a state of painful striving? The pressure builds up when you look in the mirror or nothing in the wardrobe fits and you feel the panic rising in your chest, your stomach clenching, your body stressing out.

Extending your race out to a year is like taking a big breath and as you slowly exhale, breathe out all the striving, stress and pressure you put on yourself with all its denial and unrealistic deadlines. Release yourself from that pressure. Walk away from that terrible old ineffective mental space. Give yourself permission to take the time to do the job properly.

I know we all think like the hare and want all the weight off as fast as possible but the reason I have made the Tortoise Diet Method extend over a year is that it may take time to figure out how we got into this state In the first place and you then need the time to put in place and practice the right strategies to get you out of there.

If you just keep losing kilos and then putting them back on, then it is likely that there is more to your weight gain than just over-eating.

If food is the problem, then it is likely that food itself is not the problem. What you lose in taking it more slowly, you gain in terms of sustainability. That is what we are looking for in the *Tortoise Diet Method*.

Trying to lose weight without dealing with why the weight is there in the first place is like dealing with the symptoms and not the cause. You need to get to the root cause of the problem before you can experience real and sustainable changes. It is what you do this year that will mean the difference between going on traditional type diets that you have done in the past and following the *Tortoise Diet Method*. One has brought failure and the other can bring lasting, satisfying life change. I encourage you to set aside this year to be about you – to make it your year of success. Use it to really become aware of how you got where you are today and turn that around.

You should be able to identify and then deal effectively with any issues that you discover to be holding you back. Maybe some deep issues are raised that will require the help of an expert. It is worth doing the work to get the result and now that you have given yourself time, give yourself permission to do what needs to be done.

The year will also allow you to put into practice what you are learning, gradually changing your lifestyle and environment until what works for you becomes your new familiar behaviour and is therefore sustainable. Changing your food choices gradually over time means they are more likely to last the distance. Changing your behaviour over time is more likely to become a permanent part of your life. Afterall, you have already created a normal for yourself over time that does not support your weight loss goals, so you can just as easily create another normal that will.

As you deal with what has stopped you in the past and learn new, more useful ways to live and eat, then you do what works every single day and you will get where you are going.

An important outcome of this method is that it will help you gradually adjust your baseline or your set point. Both your own comfort zone set point and your physiological set point. Everyone has a baseline, which is where our limbic system, one of those unconscious forces in our lives that you will hear more of later, has control over. It wants to make sure we maintain equilibrium in our bodies and lives. This means it has gotten used to the weight you are now and does not want it changed. Any sudden attempt to do so will end in failure, as we well know. Time can help you adjust your baseline at a pace that your subconscious can adjust to until you get to something closer to the ideal weight for you.

We all know that the more we step out of our comfort zone, the better the results we will get. However, we have also found out that the more we do that, the less likely we are to keep going so those results tend to be short term. Pushing the boundaries of your comfort zone gently and daily while gradually using the *Tortoise Diet Method* is more likely to be successful for us long time dieters. It will extend our comfort zone without our inner self getting startled by the old counterproductive behaviour of the past and then we can go on to create a new one that sustains our end goal.

Guidepost 5. The right exercise

Don't be Gym Bunny – be a gym tortoise
The same principle of going slow and steady and repeating the right actions towards the right goal also goes for exercise. You do not need to sign up for a gym membership or buy a whole lycra

kit if you do not want to, but you can get up and walk around the block.

You may find as you begin to move and discover the pleasure of a fit, healthy body that you may even begin to enjoy the challenges that gyms can offer and that the well-designed exercise clothing and shoes that we have available to us these days is something that you really want. But you don't have to start there and it's not a pre-requisite to get started on the exercise journey.

If it has been a long time since you moved, start by walking around the block or walking for ten minutes. The above principle applies. Start with what you can do and build from there, even if it is just walking for a short period. The hardest thing about exercise can be getting your shoes on but once you are out the door, the hard part is over. No one is judging you – it's up to you. The most important thing is not to approach it like the hare but more like the tortoise. You've heard of a gym bunny? Well, I suggest you become more of a gym tortoise.

> Success Work: How does it feel to get rid of those old impossible deadlines? Start thinking of the reasons you are overweight and how you can resolve them over this year.

Chapter 6

Stop Weighing Your Self-Esteem

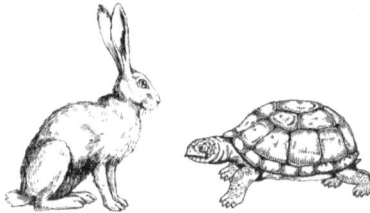

Weigh yourself once a month – if at all

Now we get to the scales! There can be a lot of fear associated with and meaning attached to what the scales say – and sometimes they even lie! Who hasn't got on the scales one day and then again the next day to find there can be a couple of kilos difference in what they read? To paraphrase Dr. Libby Weaver, it's more likely that the scales weigh your self-esteem than are an accurate reflection of what you weigh.

Most of us weigh ourselves to see how heavy we are but it is more helpful to see the scales as one indicator that measures your progress. Don't focus on the weight like you did in the old days. Remember, although the figure on the scales can be an indicator of success, it is not the only one. When approached sensibly the scales can give you feedback on whether what you are doing is working for you or if you need to make adjustments. That is how we use them in this method – not as an indicator of your self-worth.

Monthly weigh in

Weigh yourself once a month, on the first day of the month, and whatever that figure is, that will be your new benchmark. To avoid the fluctuations, always weigh yourself at the same time of the day. I suggest you weigh yourself in the morning before you have breakfast. Note that number down on the below graph under starting point. You can download a copy from the *Tortoise Diet Method* Web Page if you don't want to write in your book.

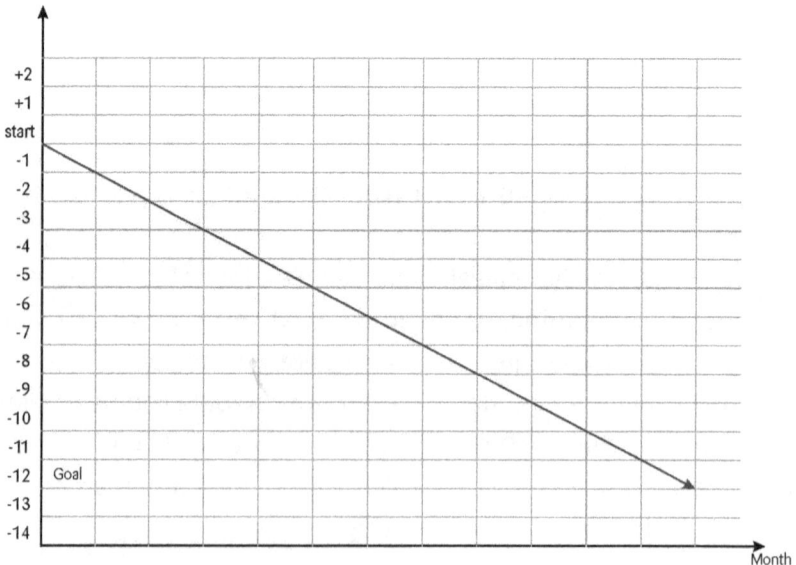

Then hold off getting on those scales until one month later, on the first day of the next month when you can weigh yourself again. Whatever that figure is, even though it might actually be more than 1 kilo, that new figure becomes your new starting point. Your next goal is to lose 1 kilo in the new following month.

For example, your start weight is 80kg, the number you weighed at the beginning of your year of success. Your intention is to lose 1 kilo a month and you get there by focusing on eating your three normal moderate sized nutritious meals a day plus the occasional extras when life calls for it and you get on and live your life.

You get on the scales the second month, and your new weight is 77.5 kilograms. So, you have lost over 1 kilogram. Well done! The new weight of 77.5 kilograms becomes the starting point for the next month and your aim is still to lose 1 kilo in that time period.

Limiting yourself to a monthly weigh-in is another way to get around obsessing with your weight. I am not a fan of scales, but as a way to measure progress and allow you to recalibrate your actions over time, they have their place. I am sure you will weigh yourself more often and it is ok if you want to do it weekly to check up on what is going on in the relationship between your new way of eating and the scales, but it is the monthly figure that counts. Avoid weighing yourself every day. That's pointless and implies the sort of disordered thinking you want to move away from.

When we look at goals in a later chapter, the aim of losing 1 kilo a month is more a key performance indicator (KPI) - than a goal. There are other KPIs you can use to measure progress that are not as emotionally loaded as the scales. You may want to take your other vital measurements (waist, hips, chest) at the beginning of your year and again once a month or so and use that as a benchmark.

Or have a nice pair of jeans or a dress that you haven't fitted for a long time and fitting into them becomes your goal. Sometimes just feeling a little more comfortable in clothes is enough for you to realise you are on the right track.

For some of us, the number that shows up on the scales carries a lot of weight – if you'll pardon the pun. I want to bring this up because this could be one of your obstacles, especially when it can mean the difference between carrying on or stopping. We can bring so much meaning to that darn number on the scales based on baggage from our long history associated with dieting. In the past, for example, when the scales didn't show regular downward losses or even showed we were putting on weight, how many of us got really discouraged and just gave up?

Fat loss is not linear. There are so many other factors involved, so don't get caught up in what the scales say. When you treat your body well, appreciating it, and giving it the nutrition it needs, it is going to go through a process of healing. Some of that work is at a deep level and not apparent to start with but keep going.

As traditional dieters, we have been too caught up in promised rapid weight loss and get very discouraged if we don't see results straight away. We are often mostly motivated (I certainly was) by appearances and expecting to see that loss showing up in our problem areas early on. So, if we didn't see those parts shrinking straight away, it was another reason to be discouraged. It may be helpful to understand that problem fat is not just hanging out annoying you on your hips, thighs or tummies. It is all around your organs as well. This kind of fat is what you want to reduce because it can be very harmful to your health. It is called visceral fat, and it is why doctors are most concerned about the weight you carry around your middle.

Visceral fat can produce certain types of proteins that can trigger chronic inflammation, putting you at risk of heart disease, diabetes, and other ailments. So even though you may not be seeing quick results, if you are following the *Tortoise Diet Method* and eating the right amounts of nutritious food for your body, then you are doing a deep work – and deep work takes time. So, hang in there and keep up the good work.

The buddy system

If you have a problem with scales, there is a solution offered in this Method. It may be that you have not really confronted the reality of how big you have become and are not quite ready to face it. Or you bring so much meaning to that starting out figure that you give up before you start. The problem I had was that if the scales showed too much success, instead of being encouraged to continue the way I was going, I would loosen up and somehow think that it was permission to eat more of the wrong things. My response was that I did not need to try so hard, so that turned into another path towards failure for me.

If any of these issues around scales are a trigger point for you, then I suggest you use the buddy system. You never have to know that figure and you won't end up giving it the power it doesn't deserve.

Get a buddy and either do the *Tortoise Diet* together or get them to be your weigh-in buddy each month. You are only going to weigh yourself once a month, let's say, on the first day of the new month. The first time you weigh yourself is merely your starting point. Get your buddy to mark that point on the graph. It's important that if the figure is higher than you expected that you don't get freaked out or reactive about it. I know that some of you will give that dratted number so much emotional meaning that you might lose the will to move forward. But it is just a number, and it is both relative and irrelevant. It is a starting point. If you think that is going to be a problem for you, get your buddy to keep it to themselves. You do not need to know what it is. All you need to know is that from this point onwards that you have lost a minimum of 1 kilo per month.

So, the only question you need to ask your buddy or yourself during weigh-in is this: Have I lost 1 kilo? It is highly likely that you have lost more than that but if like me, you have all sorts of weird responses to both too much weight loss or gain, then for the first few months it might be better not to know.

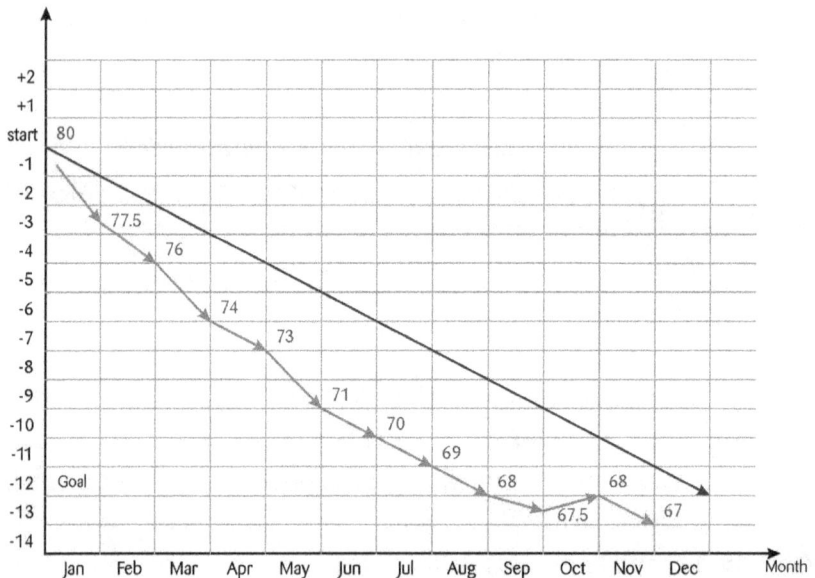

Dealing with failure – stay in the race

What happens if you do not lose a kilo? Don't panic! And certainly, do not judge, berate, abuse or punish yourself. That is something that you will stop doing with this method! But never leave the scene of failure without finding out why you failed. That way, you learn what hasn't worked and can adjust your step to what does. Turn everything into a lesson about what works for you and what doesn't.

This is your chance to take an important lesson from the fable and establish a new principle in your life that will be a key element of success. Go back to the fable and ask yourself the question; what is one thing that the tortoise did that the hare didn't do to win the race? The answer is that she stayed in the race. It just might be that staying in the race is going to be a key component of your success as you continue your journey over this year. Something we have failed to do when we have been on the old traditional type of diet.

While the hare got bored, hungry, distracted, tired and lost focus on the true goal, and basically let those obstacles prevent it from winning, the tortoise stayed in the race. That's despite the apparent physical handicaps it had, let alone all the thoughts going on inside its head! Imagine the self-talk! *I'm too slow, I'm not built for this, the hare is far quicker/prettier/more popular/got more support etc etc*. Fill in the gaps yourself. But the tortoise didn't let any of that stop her. She might have thought of them, but she kept moving despite all the obvious drawbacks and got there in the end.

The tortoise didn't let the thought of failure stop her either which it could easily have done even before she began.

Staying in the race is going to be the one new thing you are going to do that you haven't done before. Instead of giving up when you fall off the horse so to speak, get back into the saddle, learn from your experience and keep going. But this time, find out what may have contributed to what you think of as a failure and try something else.

Move away from that madness of repeating the same behaviour and towards behaviour that leads to success.

It could just be just that you ate a big meal the night before and you haven't finished processing it so you are not comparing yourself to the same situation you were in the first time around. You are not comparing apples with apples. If you are expecting to lose and haven't – just eat mindfully that day, eat enough but make sure it is light and nutritious, keep up your water intake and routine exercise up and then just weigh yourself the next day instead. What you want to avoid though, is the old behavior of yoyo dieting. You do not want to get up to the old tricks of pigging out for three weeks and starving for the fourth. That is not the *Tortoise Diet Method.*

It may sound like cheating, but we just have to move away from the rules mentality that actually leads to a cheating mentality. Cheating is something that is associated with traditional dieting. Once you figure out that you are only cheating yourself, you realise how futile it is. We already know that your weight can vary more than a kilo in a day, so remove the judgement and meaning from it and keep going. We are after authentic and long-term results here. Just keep up a steady routine and acknowledge that the scales are not always telling the full story, but they might the next day!

Now that we have that cleared up, let's go back and look at some of the other reasons you may not have lost your kilo this month.

Review the previous month. Did you loosen up so much that you had a few too many glasses of wine or a few too many treat foods over time? Do you need to up the intake of vegetables and decrease the intake of processed foods?

Have you started regular exercise and been developing your muscles? Muscle weighs more than fat, so you may not be getting an accurate reading of fat loss. We use the word weight loss when what we ideally want is fat loss. The downside and common problem with losing weight too fast on traditional short-term diets is that you lose everything but fat. You lose water and lean tissue or muscle and so while the scales show a dramatic decrease in weight, it's not the sort of decrease you want. It is false weight loss. You are after true weight loss and that may require a new mindset for you. We have all been programmed to look for dramatic results and think that if we don't get that straight away, we have failed. Again, what you are after is slow authentic re-creation of your body so that it is strong and healthy and operating efficiently – including burning excess fat.

You want to increase your muscle mass as it is muscle that burns energy. The more you have, the higher your basal metabolic rate, which is very important for true and lasting weight loss. The BMR is the rate at which your body consumes energy when you are resting – sleeping, for example. It is the basic amount of energy needed to run all the vital organs in your body and keep you alive. So quite important then. We'll talk a little more about this when we talk more about knowledge and food later, but the importance of protein in the diet will become clear.

What else? Do you need to manage yourself so that you are less stressed? Get more sleep? Has your routine been interrupted? Is it the middle of winter and you spent a lot of time sitting on the couch eating comfort food and not enough moving? Did your weigh In day coincide with your menstrual cycle? Or is your body making its own adjustments at its own pace?

Remember, our bodies are complex and don't work like machines – you could eat the same thing from week to week and your weight loss could be different if you weighed yourself each week. There is a phenomenon called a plateau effect which can happen when your body is making big adjustments over a period of time. Your weight may appear to be not moving but work is being done that you just can't see yet. Just knowing that could happen can mean you are less likely to think you have failed and therefore less likely to give up.

If you have an emotional response to not losing the amount you expected and reacted with some sort of disordered thinking - observe how that shows up. Are you catastrophising it? I have done this. Seen it as the end of the world, evidence that I am useless and a failure and that leads to eating the whole packet of whatever is around that I know I shouldn't eat but do. It is not a catastrophe. It's just a moment in time so make sure you treat it like one and stay in the race.

Making it work for you

So that's how the *Tortoise Diet Method* works. Simple but achievable. The more you are able to get into a good routine of eating from a wide variety of good whole natural foods rather than eating a lot of over processed sugar and additive laden non-foods, the more this will work for you. You will find your health improving, your mood improving, and you will start to see good changes taking place in your body. They may be small to start with but after years of failed yoyo dieting, small but sustained is good!

Never be put off by the thought of only losing a kilo or a couple of pounds a month. I am going to let you in on a little secret. I found that as I learned and put into practice these principles, that I often lost more than a kilo a month. So, it is definitely possible to lose more than just 12 kilos in a year by using this method – it's just that our diet-addled brains can get freaked out if we try to lose too much too quickly.

It seems strange that lowering our expectations helps us to succeed, but that is what we are doing. Lowering them just enough to get back into a success pattern again and allowing our bodies to reset back to a normal healthy, regular way of eating.

Once you gain confidence and get clear on what your past problems have been and have gone a long way to overcoming them, then there is no reason that you can't increase your monthly goal – but tread carefully here. Keep it at the one kilo level to start with and take everything else as a bonus – a sign that you are establishing the food foundations for a strong, slim, and healthy future for yourself.

It really all comes down to making sustainable changes and that is at the very core of the success of the *Tortoise Diet Method*. One of the real problems with traditional diets is that they are essentially unsustainable. It's all very well losing weight in the short term by 'going on a diet' but to lose it and keep it off is what we are looking for. This is where time comes into it – and why allowing yourself the time period of a year is so helpful. Let's take a look now at what to do with that gift of time.

Success Work. Use the graph in your workbook to plot your monthly weight. What other KPIs can you use? Take your measurements monthly.

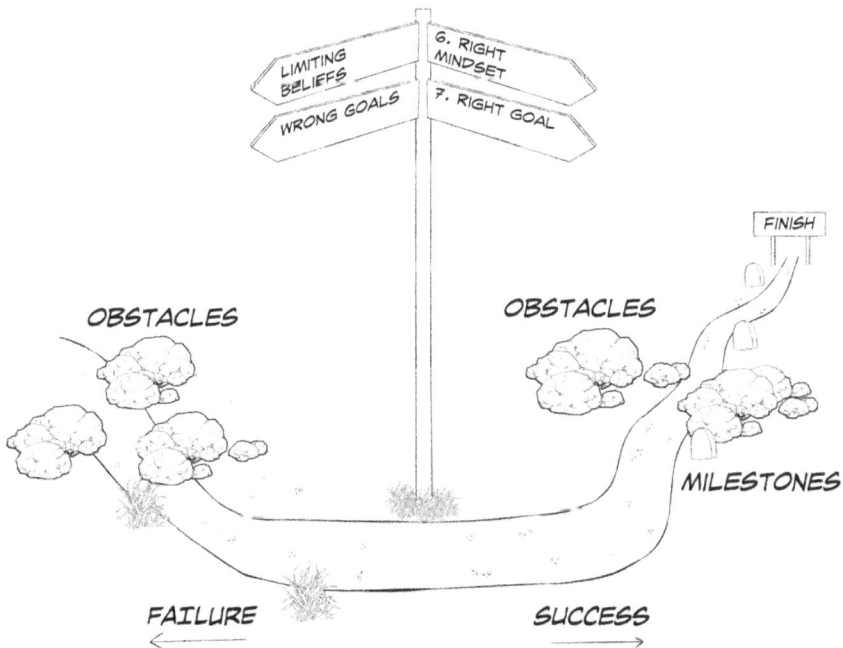

Stage 3

The Starting line

In order to win I need to be clear about where I am going and be properly equipped to run the race.

Chapter 7

Time - It's What You Do With It

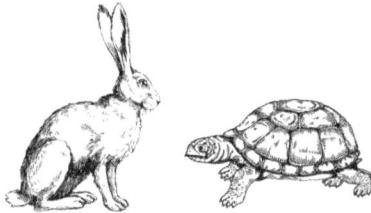

One of the most powerful lessons I have learned while developing the Tortoise Diet is to understand the concept of time. It always makes me laugh when people say they 'don't have time,' because in the end that is all any of us have. Time is going to pass whether we are aware of it or not or use it wisely or not. It may seem like a cliché, but it really is what we do with it that counts.

When you realise that the person you are today, whether it is your bodyweight, your health, your job, where you are in life or who you are with, is a result of the accumulation of the thoughts, choices and actions you have taken every single day up to this point in time, you start to get a different perspective. In a sense, we are living in our own past because we live with the consequences of the actions we took long ago. Our past can cast a very long shadow into our future when the beliefs we formed then and the thoughts we developed out of them created the habits and behaviour we live our lives in today.

For some of you, that might be a sad or painful revelation as you think of those actions and decisions that have led to unfortunate outcomes. But it is also an incredibly hopeful concept. Once we become aware of how it works we can then take a hand in working with time to go about creating the life we really want. We can learn to break free from our own history and to create that new life for ourselves by knowing where we want to go and taking daily action toward that.

It means that from this day forward, I have an understanding that what I do every single day becomes the me of the future. Time then becomes the medium I create my life in, and I create my new life by consistently taking the right actions towards my goal. As the saying goes, I may not be able to change the past, but I can start right now and build a new future. And sometimes the most important choice you can make about your future is what is at the end of your fork.

So now you have the strategy of the *Tortoise Diet Method* in place and are standing on the starting line of your race, you can begin to get your head around why giving yourself a year to do this is such a gift. How can what we do daily over the time that we have been given help us to close the gap between where we are and where we want to be? How can we deal with all the obstacles in that gap between our starting line and our finishing line – the ones that have stopped us in the past whenever we have attempted to successfully reach our goal weight?

It is during this year that you will put the time into equipping yourself for success. Everything we gain takes time; skills, knowledge, wealth, health and weight! It is going to take time to lose that weight once and for all, so giving yourself a year serves many purposes. It takes you away from the tyranny of time restriction you place on yourself. All that does is add to your stress level and keep setting you up for failure. It should also take you away from a place of striving – which is where you have been most of your dieting journey- to a place of calmness and clarity. This is a much more effective way to reach your goals.

It gives your body time to heal as you increase the amount of lifegiving whole natural foods in your daily life and decrease the ones that work against your health. As it heals, your body will be able to safely release the excess weight and get back into a natural balance that works for you.

It gives your body time to start believing that this time you really mean it – that you are not just off on another of your hare-like jaunts to lose weight again. As you consistently and daily put your new plan into action you will start to regain faith in yourself and no longer keep giving evidence to your old limiting belief mindset that you are a failure. You will daily build up a new story of success to provide evidence of your new life affirming belief that you can do this.

It is possible to make tiny changes to your behaviour each day and eventually achieve extraordinary results. A seed sown in winter can be a mature plant in summer. A seedling planted in one year can become a mighty tree in the future. You must plant the seed first, a step we often miss out, and nurture it every day.

It will be helpful to you if you can think of each day as a microcosm of your year. Like the tortoise taking one step at a time, your year can be broken down into the steps of each new day you are given. Instead of seeing your finish line as way out there in the unknown future, bring it right into your day and understand that as you eat right, move right, and think right today, you are achieving that goal. Just aim to do what works daily. When you do that, the future will take care of itself.

I think us old school dieters have made such a big thing about food that every meal is a mini drama and that is a big mindset problem for us. Once you understand it is not a drama, it is just food, and it is there to nourish you, not make you happy or feel loved or any other of those things you associate with it, then you are more likely to eat what you planned to eat and get on with more important things like living a meaningful life. After all, today will rapidly become tomorrow and then it is gone. All the angst we associate with food is no longer relevant, but what we ate will be. Make it count. Walk away from the drama!

Even though the Tortoise Diet Method is more of a marathon than a sprint, even a marathon can be made up of a whole series of sprints put together with the winning post always in mind. So if you are wondering how you can keep it up for a whole year, then there are all sorts of things you can do to keep yourself motivated. Break the year into months and have a theme or a challenge each month. If you think it's boring to eat routinely (but effectively) throughout the week, try out new recipes in the weekend and add them to your repertoire. Challenge yourself to keep up a new habit by daily marking it off on the calendar. Keep researching to find our what works for you and your specific situation. Try out new forms of exercise to find out what you like the most. Most of all, find other ways to bring joy and pleasure into your life that don't involve the counterfeit 'pleasure' of overeating the wrong foods, and enjoy and celebrate the results of a new you!

Using time as a tool

Changing our perspective on time can mean that we start to see time as a tool. What most of us have been doing over our lives is a lot of small behaviors that take us away from where we want to go. Snacking on the wrong foods, for example. Eating after dinner, even though you are not hungry – which was the bad habit that played a big part in my gradual weight gain. Just installing the new behaviour of not eating after dinner for an entire year was an important part of winning my race.

These small unconscious types of behaviour repeated daily in our lives are known as habits and they can become our secret weapon!

Habits are one of the most important building blocks of our lives. A habit is a behaviour that you once consciously chose to do (or were trained to do) then by regular and consistent repetition over time became an automatic routine. One that we no longer even think about anymore. Imagine if you could harness the power of habit over this year and create new habits that eventually became second nature, but were the ones that worked for you, not against you?

We can have good habits that work for us such as cleaning our teeth daily. That's a good example of one we have been trained to do since we were children. Our parents stood over us and forced us to clean our teeth because it was an important habit to get into to learn to care for yourself.

You can have bad habits such as eating rubbish food after dinner even though you are not hungry and don't need it. Those ones work against us. The point is that we are naturally habit-forming creatures and so it is possible to use this power for good rather than evil.

When we create those automatic behaviours, they can then become life builders that help us program our lives into reaching our goals. All of us have habits we may not even be aware of but are leading us either towards where we want to go or away from it. It is very important that we uncover and identify what they are so that we can change them to the right ones.

Putting into practise the daily habit of eating three nutritious moderate meals a day and cutting out junk food as much as you can will be a significant move in the right direction. Even if you did just that for the rest of the year, you would already be way more successful in losing weight than you probably have been until now.

Use this year to become aware of them. Observe your behaviour and become aware of the patterns you are repeating. Examine them to see if they are building the life you want or are continuing to sabotage your intention. Your habits all started somewhere with a thought or a belief before you made them part of your life. If they are no longer helpful, use this time to understand where they came from and what lies beneath your habitual behaviour. Then change them to one that does.

Equipped for success

Use this time to equip yourself for success. If you look at what you know about the tortoise, there is one thing that everyone knows

– and that is that it carries its house upon its back. It carries within it everything it needs. I'm pretty sure it is not likely to add to that – you don't see tortoises out there with a second storey added to the top of their shell, or a little trailer towing behind with extra gear. No. The tortoise carries only what it needs to get through life.

We on the other hand have acquired a whole load of baggage over the course of our life and it is that which is weighing us down and preventing us from winning our own race. It may just be that the most important organ in dealing with weight loss is our brain. It's our thoughts, the meaning we have given to things and the lies that have been told to us, or we have told ourselves and then turned into patterns of behaviour, that hold us back.

We do actually have everything we need to win the race. We were born with it – its just that with all the goings on and shouting and meaning creating and general life events that have gone on in our lives we have lost touch with that true knowing. You can do it. And it will help to lay aside the weight that has been stopping you.

Success will come over time when you require a little more of yourself. Not go crazy and suddenly make a lot of new rules and restrictions to live by as though you were on the hare diet but take on a deep, firm, calm conviction that you can break out of your old ways, that no one else is going to do it for you but with the right mindset and the right tools you can and will do it. Start by equipping yourself with a few important mindset changes to help you on your way.

A healthy sense of self-love

You would be surprised how often people who have ongoing issues with their weight have a difficult relationship with themselves and often put themselves at the very bottom of the list when it comes to being cared for. Afterall, why bother with your own health if you don't believe you are worthy? Where these beliefs come from will be different for all. Some have absorbed them from a very early age and created a whole life story around them that ends up becoming a self-fulfilling prophecy.

You do have to understand that you are loveable and learn to love yourself in order to take the steps to care for your body. I'm not talking about narcissism or selfishness but a basic understanding of your intrinsic value that is part of our wholeness as human beings.

An outcome of not loving yourself is that you neglect to make caring for your body a priority. Maybe a reason you don't stick to a good healthy diet is that you don't really believe in the importance of your own health and wellbeing. Sporadic acts of priority don't work in any area of your life. We all seem to be capable of making radical life affirming changes to the way we treat our bodies if we get a sudden diagnosis of a life threatening disease but why not start to appreciate and value your body now as the amazing piece of creation that it is? Your body is a temple – so treat the nourishing it like the sacred work that it really is.

Another outcome of valuing yourself is that you stop punishing yourself. Listen to the language around exercise for example. Have you heard of people who exercise at a "punishing" pace? And maybe you even use food as a form of punishment itself? Overeating and abusing your body by doing everything to it you know is bad for it because you feel you hate yourself is a form of punishment.

When you eat well because you value yourself you do it for you. Not to please anyone else. Of course, feeling and looking better can please your spouse or partner but pleasing them is not your primary goal. When you love yourself you look after yourself because you understand you are valuable. Becoming whole and healthy will naturally follow. For those of you out there who have tended to put everyone else before you and made yourself bottom of the care-for list, you will be much better able to care for those around you if you are well yourself. So put your own oxygen mask on before helping those around you.

You are the boss of you

Along with loving yourself another vitally important part of achieving success in this race is to update your mindset around being the leader of your own life. Ultimately, the responsibility for your life resides within you. You are the boss of you. You are no longer 18 and waiting for your mother, your school teacher or even a diet to tell you what to do or what to eat (so you can ignore it). You are responsible for yourself. Your future is in your hands. If you are overweight – the solution lies within you.

It can be tough if you look back at your life and see some of the choices that you made maybe because you didn't feel like you had a choice and how they turned out. Taking responsibility for your life and actions does not mean blaming yourself. It is not a meaning making exercise where you make a big stick and beat yourself up for all the things you did wrong and all the times you over-ate and didn't go to the gym. It definitely does not ask you to see yourself as a victim and take on that mindset.

A victim mentality can be one of the obstacles you might need to overcome if you have made a story about your life that locates blame elsewhere. Having a victim mentality can show up when we use something as an excuse to avoid doing what we know we should. It's like living with the thought police. You don't need the parent, teacher or other authority figure telling you how to run your life because you've still got their voices living in your head now telling you all sorts of nonsense.

No - in this method, you identify what some of those past actions were without judgement, without a view to recrimination, drama or punishment. Think of the tortoise as she ran her race. She didn't spend any time at all on unnecessary drama, excuses as to why she couldn't possibly do it (although she had plenty if she chose to do that) or why something that happened in her past meant she wasn't able to win. This is why I suggest you don't let your past beliefs stop you from starting the *Tortoise Diet Method*. She decided and then she did it.

Be a problem solver

The other big key for you when it comes to dealing with obstacles is to change your mindset to becoming a problem solver. Our tortoise knew there were obstacles out there, but she also knew they were not going to prevent her from reaching her goal. She had the attitude of a problem solver.

Instead of complaining about all the reasons you can't change your situation or your diet, or can't exercise, change your thinking instead. Start thinking about ways you can solve those problems. Perhaps they are not as big as when they first appeared and you will find a way around them. This kind of thinking puts the power back into your hands and makes you stronger. The power no longer lies with the obstacles as there is always a way to overcome them. The power lies with you as you learn to overcome them.

Change your perspective by changing your language. Try using the word challenge instead - or maybe even an opportunity! Adopt a growth mindset. You get stronger by overcoming obstacles and gain confidence by realizing you have the ability and power to do so. You grow in knowledge and understanding as you learn new things that you will be able to use in future to clear your path. You will also get a lot happier and a lot less anxious as you remove each source of negative thought and emotion from your life and convert them to positive ones.

Once you realise that you can overcome problems then you can commit to resolving them whether they are physical or emotional or anything in between. It takes away the time wasting we tend to do when we get stuck in losing the battle where we worry, complain about or ignore problems and therefore they continue to be the same old obstacles as before. Resolving rather than reacting to life's problems becomes the go-to action when we take on the mindset of an overcomer.

Identifying your obstacles

One of the most important things you can do with the time you have given yourself this year is to pinpoint the specific personal reasons you are overweight. Your job over the course of the year is to equip yourself with the tools to find your specific solutions to overcoming them.

There will be some obstacles that are common to many of us and some that are more specific to you. Overeating for reasons other than nourishment, such as the various forms of comfort-eating. Eating when you know you shouldn't but you can't stop. Obstacles in our environment. Lack of support. Lack of knowledge or understanding about why and how food works or how to apply it in our own particular circumstances. A medical condition. Make a list of what those are for you as you see them now.

When you understand that you are responsible for your own life you understand you will be far more effective when you find your own solutions. Sometimes you just need a bit of direction about what question to ask or what direction to go in and that is what the *Tortoise Diet Method* is about. As you work with the process yourself, you can come up with your own plan that will work for you, and you can tailor to your own specific needs and situation.

Success Work: Think about how time works. Can you think of examples of actions you have taken that have affected your life? Can you start to identify some of your habits both good and bad. Why am I overweight and what are my obstacles to weight loss? Make a list in your workbook.

Chapter 8

Goals Are Not the Goal

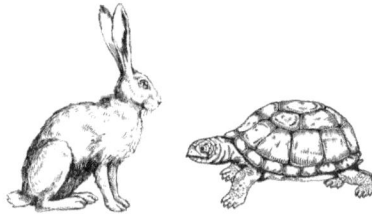

A t this stage of your race, you are standing at the starting line. You've got your new strategy to work out, you have given yourself the gift of time to resolve what has been holding you back and you are starting to equip yourself with some mindset tools for success. Now comes the time to turn your attention to the direction you are going to be running; your finishing line.

A funny thing happened to me as I thought about the finish line for my own race. I began to doubt whether I had been aiming for the right goal all along. I even began to suspect heading for the wrong goal all along was one of the reasons I had been failing in my previous attempts to lose weight. Afterall, we are always going to fail if we keep running towards the wrong goal!

If the most important part of winning any race is to cross the right finish line it therefore becomes very important to take time to make sure you are heading towards the right one. There is a very good illustration you may come across about climbing the ladder to success. You can be working away very hard putting in a lot of effort, but if your ladder is not leaning against the right wall, then you will never get the success you are looking for. Making sure your ladder is leaning against the right wall will be a key part of your success.

If I asked you what your goal was, your answer is likely to be a figure in your head that you want to reach on the scales. You see success as being in terms of losing a certain amount of weight. But what happens if you get to that goal weight and nothing else changes? We all secretly think that somehow our lives will magically transform into one of joy and happiness and all our problems will disappear when we get to that number. But what happens if you get there, and nothing has changed? What if it's not just weight loss we are really after and we have aimed for the wrong goal all along? Could that be one of the reasons we have failed so often? Too many of us have our ladders leaning on the wall of weight loss and its the wrong wall.

So what is the right finish line then? Of course, losing weight is part of it, but what you really want is what is *represented* by reaching that goal you have in your head and are looking for when you get on the scales.

So ask yourself this question instead. Who do I want to become that is represented by this number on the scales I keep trying to reach. If I asked you what it would mean to you and who you would like to become if you were at your goal weight, then you would probably have some variation of the following answer: to look your best, to feel at peace in your life, to be happy and successful, to have satisfying and loving relationship with those you love, to enjoy being fit and healthy, be full of life and energy and just show up in life the best way you can.

We all want to look good, we all want to have healthy bodies and minds, and we all want to move freely and live meaningful lives. If you are a parent, you may want to be able to physically play with your children. If you are out there pursuing a career, you want to look the best you can, be more confident and have enough energy to sustain a busy life. If you are in the older age group, you want to make sure your body is healthy so you can live out your days in a state of health and not be held back by illness.

Those are our real goals. That is why we really want to lose weight. The figure that the scales show is important only because it is one way to measure our progress towards one of the key factors of our success in reaching that goal; weight loss. The downward trending numbers are important as milestones along the way but they are not the goal in themselves.

It was Buckminster Fuller who said:

> 'You can never change things by fighting the existing reality – to change something you need to build a new model that makes the existing model obsolete'.

In a similar vein, Einstein said that:

*'You can never solve a problem using the same thinking
that got you there in the first place.'*

For much of my life, and I am going to guess for your life as well, weight loss alone was what I was striving for. What I have discovered is that a lot of things fall into place once you realise you have been in the wrong race all along and that has left you with a lot of unnecessary baggage. It is a subtle but powerful distinction. I know I am mixing my metaphors a bit here, but you need to get off that old train and get onto another one going in the right direction - and leave that baggage on the old train!

Your true goal

All of the good things we want for ourselves that we have tied up in our striving for weight loss alone, can be summed up in one word: *Wellbeing.* I think the finish line is not actually to lose weight but to *gain wellbeing*. Ironically, it is our futile pursuit of the goal of weight loss that has robbed us of much of our wellbeing.

It may take a while to make the leap in your head, but once you have made the paradigm shift, it will help stop the old striving pattern you have developed in your life. Begin to understand that you have been trying very hard all these years to do something that has been essentially impossible. Gaining wellbeing is on the other hand, very possible, and it comes with all the benefits you've been looking for all along.

The best thing about the change in focus to one of wellbeing is you will find that when you start to eat well on a regular basis, your weight will naturally balance itself out. With time and the right nutrients to do so, your important digestive organs will start to heal and function properly. Your hormones will balance out and these changes will contribute to your new healthy weight. In fact it is highly likely that you need to be well and healthy in order to lose weight! Especially in the meaningful sustainable way we are after in the Tortoise Diet Method.

This change in focus means a shift from making food choices based on calories alone - which we do when we diet – to making choices based on the nutritional value of the food so we can eat for health and wellbeing. The idea of eating for our own wellbeing, especially when we truly understand what that is for us, gives us the power to stop eating the over-processed foods we know are bad for our health but have been irresistibly drawn to in the past. It gives us the power to eat good foods without getting hung up on their calorie component.

The reason this paradigm shift is so powerful is because it gives meaning to your actions. Instead of following a 'diet' and not understanding why you are doing what they tell you to do, you are making meaningful decisions based on the outcome you are aiming for.

Look at it this way. If someone came into your room at 4am and dragged you out of your nice warm bed, made you get dressed and go out into the cold and dark and forced you to swim for two hours then train at the gym for a few more, you are going to be very resistant and do all you can to avoid it. But if you were an elite swimmer aiming to win a gold medal at the next Olympics, then that changes the meaning completely and that changes the motivation. The same thing will happen when you understand what your goal really is and why you need to reach it. The motivation will come from within and you will go from thinking in terms of restriction and denial to *choosing* what is best for you. It's the difference that comes from doing something because you choose to and doing it because you have been told to. You move from pain to pleasure once you attach the pleasure of reaching your goal to the actions you take to get there.

Being in the right race and heading for the right end goal of wellbeing makes things so much easier. All the foods that are good for you are natural, wholesome, full of colour, variety, and taste amazing. They also make you look more beautiful, give you bright eyes and clear skin, strong healthy hair, and nails, build immunity, slow down the aging process, keep up your energy, contribute to your mental health and give you a healthy self-image. What is not to like?

There are various components to wellbeing and weight is just one of them. Taking the time to really understand what you need to do to increase your wellbeing and then putting that into practice will be an important part of your journey this year.

Eating the right foods that provide the right nutrients for you, good gut health, sleeping well, exercising well, meaningful work, taking time to do things you love, having good relationships with others, and reducing stress are all components of well-being. Make learning about how to apply these things to your life be the focus of your journey.

Getting on the road to wellbeing will not only take you away from what has probably been a long and difficult relationship with food and dieting, but it will take you towards a journey of true pleasure. You will find that you enjoy food because the right ones make you feel (and look) so much better. You will enjoy moving and exercising more because it makes you feel (and look) so much better. All because you have changed your direction.

I found that in changing my focus from worrying about calories to thinking about nutrients and all the other goodies food provides, I lost that terrible nagging worry about being almost hypervigilant about food and worrying about every calorie. It meant that I lost that sense of denial or deprivation that is a fatal flaw of traditional diets. I could eat delicious food and enjoy occasional treats. It sidestepped that entire thought process – creating a whole new way to look at the problem, just as Buckminster Fuller and Einstein were indicating in the quotes at the beginning of this chapter.

Once you throw out the model that your goal is weight-loss for the sake of reaching a number on the scales and doing that by restricting and counting calories, then you also leave behind all the disordered thinking that goes along with that. Replace it with the new model – one that puts you on the right path towards health and wellbeing and all the benefits, including in the weight department. Enjoy the new freedom that brings!

Compelling vision

The goal of wellbeing is a wonderful finish line to have for your life, but it can seem a little bit generalised and maybe not exciting enough to be very inspiring at first. It is the ultimate finish line, but you need to find the way to express wellbeing as an inspirational and compelling vision, personal enough and powerful enough to keep you moving forward. That way it becomes a useful tool that you can use to not only be successful but to sustain that success.

The way to do this in practice is to turn all those things you know you want to be into your own compelling vision for yourself and your life, and then commit to it daily. Once you realise that it is *who you are going to become* when you win your race, then you realise the value of clarifying what that identity is for you. So get out your journal or workbook and take a page or two to write out what you really want. What is it that losing that weight represents for you.

Start by imagining where you want to be in your life; what is your ultimate goal – what all the factors that make up true wellbeing are for you. You can make it a specific time period like the end of this year, or 5 years, or 10 years. All will be helpful. What do you want to look like, what are you going to be wearing, what sort of person you will be, what will others say about you. Who is in your life, where you are going to be in your business, where you will live?

There are the universal goals that have already been mentioned – the ones we all want for ourselves – and then there are ones that have specific meaning for you. Note them all down in your journal or workbook. Clues can come from who you imagined yourself becoming when you were a child and before life got in the way. It may be that this new identity you are thinking of is the person you would be if all those obstacles were resolved. It might be the person you could be once you fill all potential you have.

After reading the chapter on thoughts and beliefs you will start to realise how much we have built up a whole edifice of false ones around ourselves that have prevented us from becoming that person. As we work through this year identifying and overcoming our obstacles, this new identity will be revealed. Just like the old story of Michaelangelo sculpting the angel. Others saw just a big chunk of marble. Michealangelo saw the angel within and his job was to sculpt away the stone around it to reveal what was really there. You already have this identity within you – now is the time to bring her (or him) forth.

Your vision will not only include 'what,' it will include 'why'. We all have our own reasons why we want to lose weight so put some thought into yours. You will find that some of them are push reasons. You want to move away from the negative. A heath-scare such as a cancer diagnosis is an extremely compelling reason to radically change your behaviour. You missed out on a job promotion because of your size might be another. Sometimes in your life, something happens that becomes the final straw: like being so embarrassed at overflowing the seat on an aircraft and encroaching on the person next to you that it pushes you to change your life. Push reasons can be powerful and can be the catalyst towards change, but you need more.

A compelling vision is a pull reason, one that will pull you towards it. You want to create a future so bright and beautiful and compelling for yourself that you will naturally be drawn to it and bring everything into alignment with it. The more positive emotion it inspires within you the more effective it will be.

Your thoughts may start by being a page or two long as you get them all down on paper. Then summarise it down so you can express it into one statement which will then become an affirmation that you can repeat daily. There are some important features of a truly effective vision tied up in the way our subconscious works. Your emotions need to be engaged when you are building it– which is why you want to make it so bright and compelling. You want to engage the imagination and anchor what it is creating through emotion. Emotion is the language of the unconscious so when you really feel what it's like to be that person you are aiming for, the more powerful it becomes.

When it comes to writing it down, it also needs to be written in the present tense because your unconscious acts on the information we tell it. It has a bias to make what we think and believe about ourselves to become true. So if we keep repeating to ourselves the vision in the present tense, as though we are already that person, it will do its best to make sure that statement is true. It will become our ally instead of our enemy.

Here are a couple of examples of a compelling future statement characterised in the present tense and expressed in a way that has meaning and emotion for the person who created it.

I am so amazingly healthy and gorgeous and vibrant and full of life and energy that people stop me in the street to ask me my secret; my doctor stares at my outstandingly great test results with wonderment. My husband doesn't know what I've done, but he loves the results and my family are all delighted to have a happy, healthy mum showing up in their lives.

When I choose the foods to eat that are good for my wellbeing, they make me feel so fabulous I can hardly stand it!

One of the most important things you can do towards any sort of success in your life is to know what that success is and every day, as soon as you wake up, make it a daily habit to remember, write down, repeat, visualise by using your imagination and emotion, say it out loud – whatever way you do it – make a habit of practising being that person. You can have a vision that is a few sentences long and divide it up into shorter affirmations such as the one above. Do what works for you.

Remember, our past creates our future and we have already created it unconsciously up to now whether we know it or not and will continue to do so unless we take a conscious hand in the process. Paying daily attention to and choosing our consciously created goal will go a long way to creating a different kind of future - one you have had a hand in forming.

The best way I can explain it is that by holding a compelling vision for the future and by keeping it always before you, committing to it daily, that we create the shape or mould for a new future. As we bring all of our thoughts, beliefs, actions and environment into alignment with that true goal it becomes our north star. It becomes a compass for our lives to guide us in the direction we really want to go in. That good future naturally starts to manifest in our lives – including our weight.

It is the daily practice of focusing on your compelling reason that will bring it to life. The clearer your vision is, the more compelling it becomes. What it also does is then inform our behaviour. Just like a compass, it gives us a true guide to our life, right down to what we eat. Ask yourself the question – will eating this food nourish me and take me closer to my goal? Or will it stop me from creating success for myself?

Understand that the answer is your choice and every choice you make creates your future. As you feel the positive emotions surrounding your vision, your unconscious starts to work to make what you desire a reality, and you will find many other things falling into place as well. So having a clear vision of what your goal is will take you a long way towards aligning all the parts of your life that need aligning and bring you towards success.

Goal Setting

Just because we have a new understanding of what our true goal is doesn't mean we ignore the power of goal setting and having goals along the way. Going back to our fable and ancient times, it was common on the roads to have markers at the distance of every mile, hence the name milestones. We use this word these days to mean significant markers in our lives. We reach a milestone birthday, for instance, or things like finishing your Degree, running a marathon or a similar achievement in life.

Once we think about how we set goals, it might be more meaningful to see them as milestones; markers that have meaning for us and represent genuine achievement along the way. I am going to suggest that those markers should represent a point where you have broken through a barrier you haven't been able to break through for years. For example, your first milestone could be a weight you haven't been for a very long time and if you can reach that, then you will be feel the true joy of achieving something that has been very hard to do, but you did it. Reaching a milestone in effect represents a breakthrough in overcoming very strong underlying beliefs and turning them into a new and better story; one that supports your success.

Think of what that figure is for you and write that one down. This is the one that you are going to focus on when you use the tools of daily commitment and visualisation. You know where you are starting from, make your focus the next milestone. Once there, you can set the next milestone and so on until you reach where you want to go.

Rewarding yourself for reaching that milestone is a great tool for ensuring ongoing success. A reward is something that brings pleasure and that helps our brain to anchor the positive behaviour. The trouble has been that in the past our rewards have been a big fat piece of chocolate cake! Find some others - having a bubble bath, buying yourself flowers or a magazine – something that brings pleasure but will not sabotage your gains. You could make them as simple as marking off the calendar for each day that you have repeated a new positive habit and see how long you can keep the chain going for.

I know I have just touched on some big concepts here, but I really hope that you have made an important shift in your thinking in this chapter. Walk away from the old model of endless dieting and all the baggage it brings with it. Start a new life and a new model. Focus on living your best life and allow everything to fall into place, including your weight, as you concentrate on achieving full health and wellbeing in your life.

Stage 4

Running the Race

Becoming an overcomer

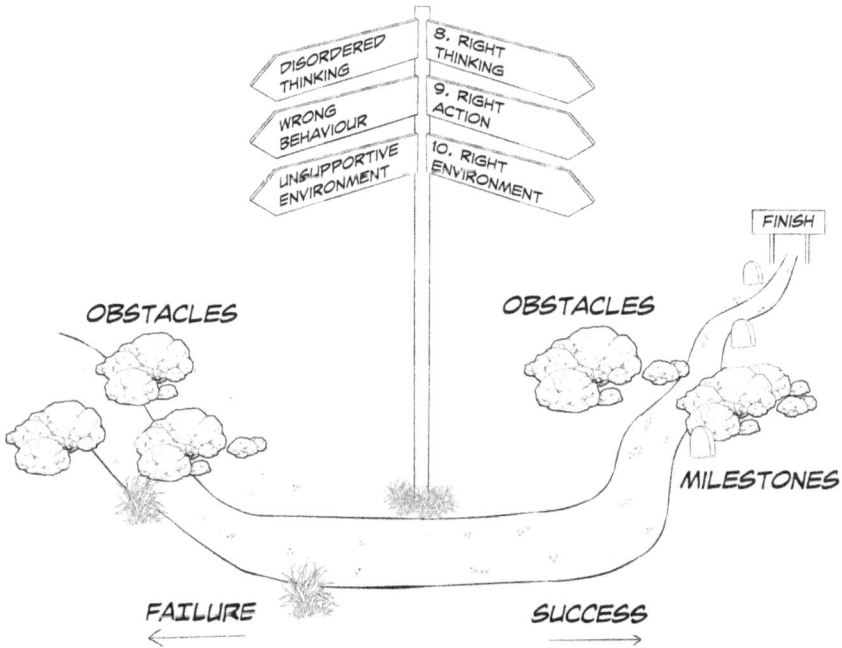

Chapter 9

What Lies Beneath

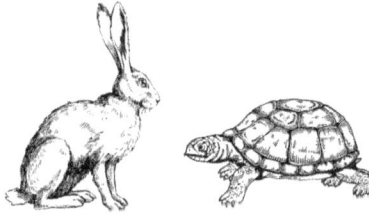

*"Until you make the unconscious conscious,
it will direct your life and you will call it fate."*
Carl Jung.

One of the great mysteries of human behaviour is this: why do we keep doing the very thing we know not to do when we are trying to achieve a particular result? Any time you do something you know is wrong, unhelpful, or not even rational but you do it anyway, you need to ask yourself what else is going on.

For us dieters this shows up in the times we eat for reasons other than nutrition such as emotional eating, comfort eating or any kind of over eating. The answer more than likely lies somewhere hidden in our inner selves, in *what lies beneath* our conscious awareness. This has probably been one of the biggest barriers to your success so finding your answer to this question will be one of the most important steps in your journey towards success this year.

There's really no escaping from the notion that your outer world is an expression of your inner world. We've already talked about how our behaviour is a reflection of our beliefs, whether we are even aware of those beliefs or not. In fact, our external behaviour will give us the clue as to what we need to straighten up on the inside. Our bodies are a mirror for our inner beliefs, and it is not just our bodies. The state of our cars, our houses, our bedrooms, our desks, wherever we show up in life, we reveal ourselves. Sometimes that can be a bit too revealing!

A good part of your year long journey is to uncover what those beliefs might be, making the *unconscious conscious* as Carl Jung says, and working to change what we find to the beliefs that are in alignment with the direction we want to go. You will have a much clearer idea of your finishing line now after doing the work in the previous chapter and you will want to make sure everything you do lines up with that ultimate goal so you can win this time round.

The journey towards weight-loss, like a lot of other things in your life, is about resolving the internal struggle before you can set about resolving the external one. Sir Edmund Hillary famously once said that he had to conquer the mountain within before tackling the one out there. There are obviously other things going on in our inner lives that are having a lot more influence on our outer selves than we might think, even though we are not consciously aware of them.

I found that over the course of the year, as I wrote and worked this *Method* out for myself this book changed from what I thought it was going to be to something deeper. My journey started off focusing on the tortoise and veered off at some stage to look more closely at the hare.

As with all myths or fables, the stories endure because they express complex truth in an apparently simple form. Which is why, of course, they speak to us so profoundly if we let them. I thought the concept of the tortoise putting one step in front of the other, over time, to reach a goal was the essence of the *Tortoise Diet* and, therefore the essence of the book. I assumed the hare was there just to provide contrast and see what happens when we do not stick to the path. But the more I pondered my own sometimes inexplicable behaviour - especially the times when I ate or behaved in ways that I knew were wrong - the more I realised that until I dealt with the inner landscape, the outer part would never change.

That inner self is represented in this story by the hare. Why on earth was this obviously talented, gifted, vibrant character who could have so easily won the race, so insistent on what was essentially self-sabotage? Why did she allow herself to be side tracked by distractions, naps, and snacks? Why the lack of focus when she knew she was in a race? Why all the talking the talk but not actually walking the walk? Why do I do all those things and why have I done all those things over a lifetime of struggle with this question?

The answer is that there is something else affecting our behaviour that we are not conscious of, and that keeps leading us to failure. Think about it this way. If you are out on the water in a kayak and want to paddle in a certain direction, your rudder needs to be aligned with that direction as well. If the rudder, which you can't see and therefore are not necessarily aware of, is jammed in another completely different direction, it's going to be very difficult, if not impossible, to get to where you are trying to go. You may even end up going round and round in circles and getting nowhere. Sound familiar?

As I took the time I now allowed myself to find what worked and what was stopping me in my own journey, I started to get an inkling of what that something else might be and where it might come from. I kept coming across the existence of this invisible world inside us that has so much bearing on our outer selves. There are whole disciplines and systems of thought and academic study around this so I am just going to touch on it here to alert you to how powerful an influence *what lies beneath* has over you. This will go a long way to helping you understand the mystery of self-sabotage: that mysterious behaviour that stops us making changes to our behaviour even when they are good changes!

There are many variations for the names and distinctions for this inner world. Call it the subconscious, the unconscious, the limbic or nervous system, the inner man or the old man (woman), the inner child, the old brain, the ego, the super ego and so on. You just need to know that somewhere in our inner self, we can have an invisible underlying belief that keeps running a program, just like a hidden piece of software on a computer, that is the real reason we cannot seem to get our behaviour lined up with our perceived goal.

Just like the invisible rudder on our kayak, it keeps taking us to where it thinks we should go not where we think we want to go. The trouble is, that program was created long ago when we were not even necessarily conscious of our thoughts, only our emotions and feelings, and since it is primarily concerned with our safety and protection, it set up a self-protection system at a very fundamental level.

Something happened to us that interrupted our perfect world and in order to make sense of this trauma, meaning was put around that event and a perception was created. That perception then coloured our thoughts and our thoughts shaped our beliefs, our beliefs turned into our actions and those actions were repeated over time to become our behaviour. Since it is our behaviour that ultimately shapes our lives, it is our behaviour that produces the results we have in our lives now.

This is all the work of perhaps the most powerful force that lies beneath; our subconscious. It is the innate force designed to keep us alive and it can have an awful lot to say in our how we behave without us realising it.

Putting it simply, there are different parts of our brain that operate in different ways and even in different time frames. One part is referred to as the old brain, which is where our automatic responses are controlled from, the ones that keep us alive and which we hold in common with other mammals. Then we have the distinctively human parts of the brain; the frontal lobes, which is where the more recently acquired logical and rational parts of us are located and we are conscious of.

This old brain controls all the automatic things such as breathing, digestion, healing wounds, growing hair and fingernails, etc through the limbic system. It oversees maintaining our setpoint through the process of homeostasis to keep returning us back to our equilibrium or what is normal or comfortable. Incidentally, this setpoint applies not just to our body systems, but to our emotional state and beliefs, which may explain why it is so hard to change our ways in many areas of our lives. All of this happens subconsciously – we don't need to think about it.

The subconscious is primarily concerned with keeping us alive and safe. It does this through the tools of instinct and emotion, including the fight-or-flight response. When it comes to keeping us safe from danger, no distinction is made between whether it is from a sabre tooth tiger or a stressful life situation, you need to be ready at any moment to get out of danger. There is no time for thought, you just need a massive dose of adrenalin or cortisol to get you out of whatever that danger is perceived to be. When it comes to a competition between the subconscious and the conscious brain, it is the old brain and its powerful goal to keep you alive that is going to win over rational thought every time.

This invisible force is essentially running that program way beneath your conscious mind, with your very best intentions and indeed, your safety in mind, but it is at odds with the new thoughts and intentions you want in your life now. Safety first!

For instance, not only does our old subconscious brain want us to keep safe, it obviously doesn't want us to starve. So, if there is even a whiff of going on a diet, restricting or cutting calories, that can be interpreted as famine approaching. It is no surprise then that you have activated the old brain which just thinks you are crazy to stop eating because food is the fundamental thing that keeps us alive. You can only then get so far into a drastic diet before this system kicks in and triggers the urge to quickly eat everything we see and then some. Which explains why I often had what I called an equal and opposite reaction the times I tried dieting.

No wonder we develop disordered thinking over the years when all of that is going on underneath. This is one of the reasons the *Tortoise Diet Method* is so effective. There is no drastic change. When you allow yourself to eat plenty of nutritious food there is no indication of lack so the warning system is bypassed. This way you can sneak under the radar of that old limbic system!

Remember also that we talked about the reason we fail at diets when we move too quickly away from what is normal. That's another function of our subconscious. Safety in the old days came from what was familiar and danger from the unfamiliar so it's no wonder diet behaviour is sabotaged when you change your eating patterns suddenly.

By starting where you are with your normal food patterns (familiar) and then gradually incorporating new nutritious foods in the right proportions (unfamiliar) so that they eventually become familiar you are working with your natural human behaviour rather than against it. And by doing this gradually over time, you don't alert all the troops in your inner world who hate and fear change.

Limiting beliefs

This subconscious programme will also show up when we have a deeply held unconscious belief that conflicts with our conscious belief – or the new ones you are wanting to create. You want to lose weight, but somewhere deep inside, you have another invisible but limiting belief that says something else. *You are not good enough. You don't deserve it. That's for other people. Being fat protects me from having to form a relationship*. The problems that result from the limiting beliefs of not valuing yourself or not believing you have power over your own life are two we touched on in an earlier chapter.

These beliefs have developed in response to a painful event in your life and are designed to protect you from future pain or danger. While they may protect you on some level, they do not serve your new intentions. You will get some sort of payoff from the behaviour that results from these beliefs, but they are keeping you locked into failure.

As we grow from tiny babies into childhood, this deep invisible part of us interprets the world in a certain way; a way that helps to make sense of life and to provide protection in the future should that situation arise again. It gives those events meaning in order to make sense to them and that shapes our perception of the world. This process does not even have to be in words or involve thought. The information absorbed by the child is more the language of emotion. Being surrounded in love and abundance, as opposed to anxiety, fear or feeling of lack, can speak to the very young through the energy of the emotion that surrounds it. This is safety at its core level. After all danger can come from an anxious, angry parent as much as from a sabre tooth tiger.

As we grow, we continue to lay down beliefs from our interpretation of the things that happen to us and what our parents, teachers or the bully in the playground say which we receive when we are in a highly vulnerable emotional state. These messages can be positive or negative and even though we may not be aware of them, they have a great bearing on the outcome of our lives. They could even be something that an authority figure said in the moment without realising the power those words had over you or having any idea of your highly emotional state at the time. Those beliefs then become the fundamental way we show up in the world, even though we may no longer be conscious of them.

The problem is that those beliefs stay on well past their use-by date and end up becoming what is commonly known as self-limiting beliefs. You've all heard the story about the elephant at the circus tethered by a tiny stake and chain even though it has the strength to pull it out in an instant. Why doesn't it just pull up the stake and then be free? Because it believes it can't do it based on the repetition of experience when it was young and weak. When the elephant was a baby, it was tethered the same way but did not have the strength to pull them out back then. Every time it tried, it could not do it until eventually it gave in and gave the power to the tiny stake and chain holding its now adult self in.

Having a good understanding of our emotions, which we understand through pain and pleasure, and how they work, will be helpful here. Our emotions also originate to a certain extent in this old brain part of us and were an important tool for survival. The urge to move away from pain seems very sensible when it comes to survival and so the move towards pleasure seems to make sense. When we experience good pleasurable things, we obviously want to repeat them and when we learn what to do to avoid that which is dangerous and painful, we also want to repeat. The role of emotion is to anchor that knowledge and makes us remember those times so we can repeat them automatically without thinking and therefore stay safe.

That's why trauma in childhood can affect us. A message is received when we are in a highly emotional state, and it sticks. It is also the reason emotion is a key to anchoring new beliefs, such as your own compelling vision that you are aiming for. The more positive emotion you give to that new vision for your life, the more you are speaking the language of the subconscious and bringing it into alignment with your goal.

The subconscious naturally uses the feelings of pain and pleasure to control our behaviour, and this is a useful tool to consider when we want to be successful on the *Tortoise Diet Method*, especially if we struggle with emotional eating. Consider that one reason we have put on weight in the first place is that we get a distorted idea of what genuine pleasure is. We have created substitute ways to get pleasure when we feel in in some kind of pain – often emotional pain. We go into child mode and feel that eating those sweet things that comforted us when we were children will help. But we don't stop at a couple of chocolate biscuits or one bowl of ice-cream. We eat the lot.

Does that produce pleasure? No. It leads to pain. This is a distortion of our natural pain-pleasure response and a common reason behind our diet failure. We can feel pain because we are over-hungry as well and if we have developed a distorted relationship with food over time, plus the added layer that comes because we have restricted ourselves, our response is to over-react and overeat - which leads to pain. So, the cycle starts all over.

The trick is to retrain yourself as to what genuine pleasure is so you can change your behaviour. I've invented my own scale which I call the Scorched Almond Continuum. Scorched almonds are my favourite chocolate treat and I have had lots of empirical evidence to support this concept.

Scorched Almond Pain/Pleasure Continuum

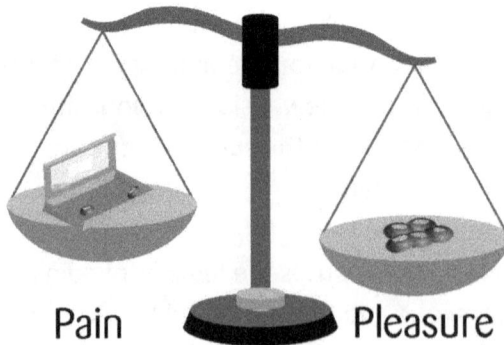

Pain   Pleasure

I ask myself the following question: how many scorched almonds can I eat before I go from true pleasure into pain? Maybe five maximum? So I allow myself those five, one at a time and really savour them. Then stop because I know that the scale will tip over into pain after that and get increasingly painful if I keep going and eat the whole box. (again – I have direct experiential proof of this).

Apply the same process to any other area of weakness you have. How many glasses of wine? It all gets blurry after a couple, doesn't it and is that really pleasurable? How much more wonderful life is when we experience true pleasure and not the old lies of pain masquerading as pleasure.

Stop and think about what true pleasure might be when you are trying to avoid feeling the pain of emotional upset, boredom, procrastination, or any other form of pain you have in life that has triggered overeating before. This natural desire to move away from pain and towards pleasure can then become a powerful tool to deal with these kinds of situations. Start to link painful emotion to those old reward behaviours. Remind yourself how terrible you feel when overeat. Replace it with an alternative behaviour that will be both pleasurable and take you closer to your goal, and then apply pleasurable emotion to that new behaviour. It will take time, but it works.

Bear in mind that this may work best when you literally take yourself out of the environment where the trigger to overeat is occurring. You can then put yourself into another state by doing something different, something that brings pleasure but a different sort of pleasure to the old destructive false one. One that works for you and not against you. Going for a walk. Taking some time for yourself. Read a book. Have a bath. Clean a cupboard. Link pleasure and positive emotions with those new behaviours. Come up with a list of those better behaviours so you are prepared. Replace your old false pleasure rewards with true pleasure ones and see how your life changes.

There is another characteristic of the subconscious that has held us back in the past, but we can turn around to help us succeed. That is its bias to make what we say to be true. It was not just the words that others said about you that affected you in the past - you must watch what you say to yourself today. Words carry power and meaning – including your own words.

If you often say, for example, that you hate exercise, then your subconscious goes about its business making that statement to be true. It activates all the unconscious commands for you to lie down on the couch until the thought of exercising goes away. That is why so many of us don't go to the gym even when we have paid our dues. You can either beware the self-fulfilling prophecy of your spoken and unspoken words or use them to your advantage.

Of course, you don't need to become an expert or know all about what lies beneath in order to succeed on the *Tortoise Diet Method*. You just need to understand that there are other forces within that shape your behaviour. This understanding first relieves you from always blaming yourself and thinking you are going crazy for repeating behaviour that not only seems irrational but is downright dangerous to your health. It then gives you the power to use our natural basic human tendencies to shape the behaviour that we need to reach our goals.

Making the invisible visible

The clue to finding out if you have an underlying belief that is at odds with the direction you want to go in is found in your behaviour.

It shows up in your actions, your emotions, and your language – even your dreams. It can reveal itself in your body – in your weight, your health, or the way you breathe.

Have you ever thought about the saying that you vote with your feet? You stop calling the person. You stop going to that job. You don't show up. You stop going anywhere that you deep down and maybe even not consciously know that you don't want to go. This is your actions revealing your inner beliefs. Pay attention.

They also show up in the gap between what we say we value and what we show we value. We may place our personal health and wellbeing high on our lists of what we value in life, but has your behaviour shown that to be true?

How is your breathing? Do you breathe deeply and regularly or are you shallow breathing and taking small quick breaths? One is telling your subconscious you are safe and that there is no danger so it doesn't have to keep pumping cortisol and adrenalin into your system just in case you need to get out of danger really quickly. The other is signalling to your body that danger is imminent so keep on high alert – and keep those hormones pumping! Slowing down your breathing and taking a few deep breaths will speak safety to your unconscious self.

Once you understand the powerful invisible forces behind why we behave like we do, whether it's the subconscious old brain, the unconscious patterns that we share with all humans that make us human, or the particular way we have viewed the world that has led to the stories we create and live from, then we can set about actively changing them. It also should change your perspective and approach to the way you have behaved in the past when it comes to dieting. Now you see that behaviour as the visible manifestation of the invisible belief, and you can now deal with it.

It can take a little bit of work to uncover some of the more deeply held invisible beliefs that have had such an influence on your life. They tend to hide in your blindspots, your avoidance behaviours, your confusion and resistance – and in the particular obstacles that you throw up in your own path. You may want some extra help in this area and I am sure it will be worth it if you do.

Updating limiting beliefs

It can be possible to update that software program running beneath your life. Identifying them is the first step. For the most part you start the change yourself by becoming aware of what you 'always do' when you go on a diet but get stopped. Listen to your language and start to notice when you repeat words about yourself that reflect a core but limiting belief. Notice your patterns of behaviour. What do you do repeatedly without even thinking that Is making you put on weight?

Once you become aware, whether it is an outward behaviour or you catch yourself going down an old negative inner thought pathway, stop what you are doing. Then interrupt the action. Go to your pre-prepared list of other things you can do to reward yourself that doesn't involve mindlessly eating sweet treats. This is a version of changing your state – it is your emotional state that can so often lead us to these negative places so breaking that pattern will be key for you. Or go to your list of new positive beliefs and stories you have made about your life and replace the old one with the new. Make them positive and in the present tense. Then as you catch yourself thinking old thoughts and patterns, stop and go down a different new life affirming thought track – one that you prepared earlier.

Keep practising this new behaviour until it becomes your new familiar and the building block for your new life.

The power of habit

I hope that you can now see some of the reasons you behave in certain ways. The problem is that some of these behaviours have turned into habits that you are no longer even conscious of. The thing about habits is that they really are the building blocks to life. Creating habits is something else the unconscious is good at because it saves a lot of time and effort. If habits have built your life and some of them have not been good for you – then why not harness the body's natural habit-forming tendency to create some good ones!

There are two components to creating habits. The cue; something that triggers the habit, and the reward; the pleasure or payoff that comes from completing it. You might come home after a hard day at work. It's a horrible old night. You are feeling tired and cranky, and your regular drive takes you past a certain fast-food joint. Now this outfit is way more skilled and knowledgeable about this sort of science than you and has trained you for years that when you see their symbol, that it is the cue that you can come in for some instant pleasure. You stop and fill up with fast food.

By the time you get home, you are not hungry and don't eat your dinner, or you carry on and eat the dinner anyway because you feel guilty about the side-trip and want to cover your tracks. Trouble is, if you keep feeling the way you do, keep driving home the same way, keep getting triggered by the sign, and keep getting the reward, then it is not long before that has turned into a habit. And if you keep eating two dinners, one of them being highly processed and unhealthy, then it's no wonder you have put on weight.

The fact that you are not experiencing the true pleasure that comes from waiting that little longer and enjoying a home-cooked nutritious meal because you have a good appetite does not come into it. When it comes to habits, reason is not always involved. It might have been way back in the beginning when you formed those habits, but is that reason past its use-by date and do you need to update it? The example given above is a good example of how much your environment can contribute to weight gain. We have triggers all over the place to behave or eat in ways that do not serve our long-term goals.

During this year, try to notice your habits, which you will probably identify in your patterns of behaviour. Examine them to see if they are building the life you want or continuing to sabotage your intention. If they are not helpful, use the time to understand where they came from. Somewhere in the past, there was a cue that led to some sort of payoff. Did you develop that habit because of a long-gone defence response to something that happened to you when you were a child? Something that happened in the past that is now having an unnecessary effect on your future?

We have habits of thought as well. Our thinking can have long ingrained paths it follows and therefore we end up in cycles of defeat. For example, you may overeat one day and that triggers a pathway of thinking the sort of thoughts that are critical and abusive towards yourself. Doing that repeatedly creates neural pathways in your brain that are just as real as the ruts created on the earth of a well-worn road. If you are a skier, think of the tracks created in the snow at the top of the run where all those who have gone before you have been. It is just a lot easier to go down the track of least resistance, the one that is familiar, the one that has become a habit. And we do that with our thoughts and behaviour daily.

That could well be one of the obstacles in your life that has prevented you from winning. It is possible to change those habits and, in fact, you will need to in order to break free and reach your goal this time. The science of habits shows that you can build new habits by finding the right trigger and using the power of reward. We gravitate towards those diets that promise instant results, and some of you get on the scales every day. You are looking for that reward that says – yes! You have lost something! Because we are looking for slow and sustained results with the *Tortoise Diet Method,* you will not get that sort of instant feedback reward. The reward needs to be close to the behaviour – we can't really handle delayed gratification when it comes to installing new habits. So, figure out a way that you can get some reward from eating in this way.

I make it a practice when I lie down at night to notice how good I feel after successfully following the method like I should. If I've eaten well, have not overeaten, have not eaten some processed food that does not agree with me, have been for some exercise, etc. It is surprising how well you will feel very early on. It's like a little bit of wellbeing in the form of a daily dose that is the promise of what I am going to feel when I succeed. This is a true form of pleasure.

Another reward that you can use it to cross off the day on your calendar. This is a way to visually map your journey. It's even better when you know that you have done well that day. I also love waking up the next morning and feeling a slight 'empty' feel, as though I provided my body with exactly what it needed to work properly and use what it needed to run my healthy metabolism from my fat stores rather than anywhere else.

Changing habits requires effort and discipline to begin with but will get easier and then eventually become second nature. There are many theories that say how long it takes to install a new habit so see what works for you. That's the beauty of allowing yourself time.

The power of the story of the Tortoise is tied up in the power of taking the right steps daily. Finding out for yourself what those right steps are for you and then making them into habits will be one of the best ways to do that and as you work through the next few chapters, turn what you have learned into a new life affirming habit.

Success Work: Put these new beliefs into practice by doing something daily to reinforce them as new habits. Do something to show yourself or your body that you love it. Practice being a leader in your own life by stepping up and doing what is right rather than what is easy. Practice overcoming by doing something daily, no matter how small, to get into the habit.

Chapter 10

Be The Boss of Your Environment

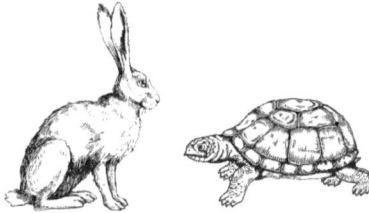

Now we can get into some more practical steps to set you up for success. You will find this a lot easier as you change up your limiting beliefs and replace them with the ones that align with your goal. You will start seeing this work itself out in your external world as well.

Do you realise that you have created an environment around you that supports being overweight? The more overweight and the longer and more chronic you have lived like that, the more you have set up the environment to support it. This goes for your inner world and your outer world.

It goes from what food you have in the fridge and the pantry, to how you shop, to who you hang out with, and how you spend your time. It also includes the books and magazines you read, and the TV shows you watch. It includes the environment in your head and all the thoughts you think, the chatter that goes on in there, and which parts of that you feed.

It is not just the food you need to manage when it comes to your weight loss, because it's not just food that has made you fat. This is one of the main reasons we could not stick to a diet in the past. We have only seen it as being about making a lot of changes to what we eat and maybe to exercise, but then we continue to live in the same environment that made us fat in the first place.

How is your lifestyle set up to support being overweight? Do you have a pantry full of tempting treats readily accessible when you feel the urge to nibble? Do you shop when you are hungry? Do you have a shopping list that includes what you need to create the meals that make up your daily steps to success? Or do you never plan your meals so that when you get home from a hard day at work, you eat everything in sight and your desire for ordered steady weight loss goes down the tube?

Are your running shoes or exercise clothes hidden away and take more effort to access than the urge to get out and exercise? Do you have no time in your schedule to walk or go to the gym or do a form of exercise that you like? Do you park as close as you can to work so you don't have to walk too far? Do you take the lift or the steps? Do you make excuses as to why you can't move your body?

Who do you hang out with? Do you have a bunch of friends who are all on the same wavelength as you in whatever addiction or negative behaviour you indulge in? When you get together, do you all support each other in bingeing on junk food, alcohol, watching junk TV or talking about unimportant things?

Who do you look up to? Do you really believe that the celebrities look like they do without a lot of interventions that are not available to you? Do you live on a diet of junk magazines and junk role models? If so, consider that the messages being sent to you are false ones that will set you up for ongoing failure.

Is your lifestyle full of a sense of overwhelm, always busy, always behind the eight ball, always rushing and stressed? Do you have time for yourself to feed your soul, to feed your desire to want a better way to be in the world? Do you have time for all the things you know contribute to the sort of wellbeing you really want for yourself?

Or do you feed your body with what are really counterfeit ways to bring relief from all that pain? Look at how you live your life. Where are you vulnerable or at your weakest?

Creating the right environment for success goes hand in hand with the creation of habits because habits are triggered by cues in the environment which sets automatic behaviour into action. If we use the earlier example of your commute home after a hard day at the office which takes you past the local fast-food joint which triggers the cue to pop in and have pre-dinner meal, then changing your environment to avoid the trigger is one way you can avoid the habit.

As we learned in the section under habits, it is the cue /reward setup that is the powerful component of habit forming. If there is no cue, the habit is less likely to roll out automatically. Try changing your journey home from work so it does not take you on that route. Changing your patterns or routines is a good way of interrupting the old ways and rethinking and re-evaluating what you are doing.

How does your environment, the way you think, the way you set up your home, your office, your personal life, who you hang out with, how you spend your time, support you in your journey to this beautiful new you? And how can you reshape your environment so the cues and triggers set you off on the sort of automatic habitual behaviour that works for you – not against you?

Be the boss of you

This is where we can try on the mindset of being the boss or manager of our own lives and start managing our environment for success. Think of yourself as not just a manager or boss of your own life, but in having agency and being the co-creator of that life. Take some leadership in your own world and turn it into one that supports everything you need to become well, whole, and successful in reaching your goals.

When you think of your environment, think of it in terms of the backdrop you live your life against, as if you are the artist or author and you are placing yourself in your own story. Once we realise we don't have to be victims of our environment but have a hand in creating it, we are on the way to a much better and more successful life. How can you, as the boss, the manager of your environment, create the sort of life that makes it easy for your compelling future vision of you and your life to come true?

There are several important roles for a manager of a business:

- Provide direction and leadership.
- Look for risks before they happen.
- Create systems to increase efficiency.
- Ensure the well-being of everyone in the company.
- Ensure you reach your goals.

Part of a manager's job is to scan the horizon looking for trouble so you can minimise risk. You are then prepared for it when it happens or can take action to prevent it from happening. I can't believe I never clicked on to that before when I kept failing at dieting. I was stopped by the same obstacles every time. You would have thought I would have no longer been surprised when it happened again and somehow thought of coming up with a plan to counteract it. That's one good thing about being an experienced dieter. We should have a good handle on what the obstacles are that stop us and therefore, with our new mindset and approach, work out a way to overcome them.

If I know the obstacles that are likely to come up then I can be prepared for them. Think ahead and plan a course of action for when that happens. Role play the various scenarios that could occur and how you, as the manager of your life, would handle it. How can I manage my environment so that I avoid the old triggers and the old patterns of behaviour and what can I do to support and reinforce the new ones? What do I know about my life and what obstacles can I predict that with a little organizing I can successfully overcome and even possibly make disappear, so they are no longer an obstacle? Wouldn't that be great?

The other part of a manager's job is to get organised and put systems in place to make sure that as much of your life as you can control runs smoothly and easily, and ideally automatically, to take you to your goal. Planning and creating systems in your life are keys to success in any area.

Let us start with something simple and obvious and located in your kitchen. You are going to be more successful in setting out to achieve your goals if you have the right foods available to eat every day and the less helpful foods less accessible in case of the more vulnerable moments. We eat with our eyes. Just seeing the trigger foods can make it so much harder to not eat them. What we think we want to eat or 'must have now' to eat is shaped by what we see. So, either don't have them, hide them or make it very hard to access them if you must, so that by the time you find them, the urge has passed.

Having the right foods available will require some reorganizing in your pantry and fridge. If your weakness is chips and you have a shelf full of them in your pantry, then get rid of the ones you have on the shelf. Same goes for sugary treats that will tempt you. And by getting rid of them, I do not mean eating them all yourself, so you do not 'waste' them! If you feel the urge to do that it could point to a problem belief. Remember – your body is a temple, not a rubbish bin or a trash can. Love and value yourself enough not to treat it like a trash can by eating trash to avoid waste.

Once you have aligned your actions with your goal of eating for you and your family's health and wellbeing, then you are more likely to have your fridge and pantry full of healthy and satisfying foods. You might as well teach your children from the start to know how much better we feel when we eat good, wholesome food and treats that don't mess around with our hormonal systems and make us sick.

You all know about the advice that if you are trying to break free from an alcohol addiction, don't go to the pub. Stay away from the triggers that create the old environment that supports that. Don't keep a house full of wine if you are trying to give up wine.

Lift your game

How are you spending your time? Watch what you watch. Is it building you up or keeping you where you were? Lift your game. Set your sights a little higher.

As part of cleaning up your environment, you may change where you hang out and who you hang out with. Who are you hanging out with in your down time? Are they supporting your new behaviour or are they just your 'friends' because you can all comfortably indulge in over drinking, overeating, over smoking or whatever it is you like to overdo that is not working towards your new life? Chances are that it is very hard to go and hang out with them without doing any of the above because you associate that environment with all of those things you no longer want to do.

The other thing is they will never hold you to account for your behaviour. So, they are enabling you to stay where you are. Do you really think those friends will support you if you decide to take the actions to turn around your life and make the changes necessary to get to the weight you desire? Of course not. They are going to do everything they can to keep you on the same level as them.

I know this sounds harsh and you will need to work out a way to manage that in terms of friendship, but if you are seriously wanting to succeed, there will be some difficult steps you may need to make to program your world for success. Often these people are not actually your friends at all, they just share an enjoyment in a certain behaviour. Once you stop that behaviour you may find there is nothing left in common. They could be threatened by you wanting to change your behaviour. They may see it as a reflection on them and their own inability to grow and change. On the other hand, true friends will love you and support you in your growth.

Of course, it's not just food that has led to us being overweight. Can you manage your environment in terms of your perception of stress?

Caring for your wellbeing becomes very current when you think how much stress is such a common theme in the modern way of life and can be the thing making your fat. Deadlines, problems at work, too much to do, fear about health, wealth, our children, our parents, whatever it is for you, are perceived as a threat by the limbic system and your fight-or-flight response is activated. What stress does is stimulate adrenaline production, which our very clever bodies think we need in order to escape the sabre tooth tiger or whatever the particular danger was when we still lived in those halcyon days of long ago. Now, of course, stress is all pervasive and never goes away. Therefore, neither does the natural biochemical response to stress – adrenaline.

So how does this affect our weight? Well, the adrenaline tells our body that it needs to move fast, so just use that glycogen that's right there, readily available as your fuel to get the heck out of there. Fat takes longer to access, so is less available in an emergency.

If you are in a chronic state of stress, then it is likely you are also in a chronic state of raised adrenaline levels and you are literally training your body to use its glucose reserves rather than the fat reserves that you have plenty of and would really rather your body used up!

Now here is the tricky bit. You've used up your reserves and now your biochemistry wants to top up those reserves, so it sends the message to your brain that you need more sugar. Hello sugar cravings. And that is a very simple explanation of one of the ways it happens.

Managing stress in your life will go a long way toward managing your weight as well as your wellbeing. Look at your life like you are a good manager and avoid being tired and stressed. They both lead to overeating behaviours. Delete, delegate, and decide to live your life differently. Factor in downtime and recreational time in your schedule.

Breathing properly (diaphragmatically) and meditating are both ways to let your subconscious know it is safe because you cannot be physically able to breathe slowly and deeply if you are on the run. Therefore, the subconscious limbic system assumes you are safe and don't need any extra help to get out of there. Practising good breathwork is a way to manage stress. Changing your perception of what is stressful may help. Stress to one person is a challenge for another. Listen to what you say, do you often talk about how overwhelmed or how stressed you are but cannot seem to do anything about it? If you value yourself, make the necessary changes to your environment around stress, including getting some professional help if necessary.

Getting organised

"Planning is bringing the future into the present so that you can do something about it now." Alan Lakein.

The more organised you are, the more successful you will be. When it comes to mealtimes, eating the right food regularly is one of the key steps to reaching your goal. Get yourself organised and prepared so you have everything you need to hand. It will help you reach your goals more than just about anything else. Plan a menu for the week– or if that seems too hard, at least plan what you are going to eat today.

Planning is a management tool that helps you to prepare for what you know is going to happen, so think ahead and work out ways to deal with situations you think may be tricky.

One tool that is very useful, especially for a busy family, is to rotate meals on a weekly or fortnightly rotation. I bet no one will ever notice, especially if you take the time on the weekend to try out a new recipe on the family or yourself and then, if it works, that can be added to the pool. I write out all my 'go to' recipes on an index card with a list of ingredients on the back so if I plan for a week or fortnight, I can just check the back of the card to add anything I need to the shopping list. I then file those cards in an index box under the days of the week they are going to be cooked.

You can get the family to help choose one and then help make it, or you can just make an executive decision. Whatever you do, make sure that you plan it and then eat what you have planned. You would not normally be able to do this on a traditional diet, but the whole point of the *Tortoise Diet Method* is that you eat with the family. Just make sure that your meals are made up of the good foods your body needs.

Cooking a little extra may mean you can eat well for lunch the next day. Make sure you have sandwich fillings and salad available. Individual pots of muesli, fruit and yoghurt. Prepare the following day's food the night before. Have containers available to make up meals so you can have food ready when you need it. Snacks included.

Have supplies of boiled eggs ready, or small containers of nuts or cheese ready for your afternoon snack. There is a bit of psychology going on there too. It helps with hunger management to know the food is there when the right time comes to eat it. Eliminate risk wherever it is.

Same for exercise as for food. Make sure your walking clothes and shoes are ready for you in the morning, so you don't have to spend fifteen minutes looking for everything. As an example, I love walking. It is a great option as it's something that we can do just about anywhere we are on earth. I am an early riser who used to spend most of the workday sitting on my bottom in front of a computer, so a walk in the morning before work is a good option.

The problem? It was often still dark, and I didn't want to disturb the sleeping husband beside me by turning on the light, fossicking through the drawers to find the right socks or loudly saying rude words when I couldn't find my shoes.

The solution? Get everything ready the night before and put it somewhere that I could find it without tripping over, turning on the light, or searching for my clothes and shoes. I even progressed from there to putting all my exercise clothes, socks, hat etc., in a special bag in my closet and making sure my walking shoes had their own home and always lived there. I could just grab the bag and go out to another room to get ready. Minimal disturbance, minimal time wasting and maximum result. A small example I know, but don't let the problems that stopped you before put you off now.

The biggest lesson we are looking for here is to be prepared for what lies ahead, both the known and the unknown.

Managing your internal environment

Managing your internal world is going to be a key part of your journey. Rationalising your life, reducing stress, focusing on the meaningful activity, getting rest, and restoring your soul are all steps you can take towards keeping in the best state for success. We all know that it is when we are down, depressed, under pressure, tired or overwhelmed that we are most vulnerable to the behaviours that don't serve our best selves. So, while our invisible and unconscious thoughts and beliefs influence our external environment, it works the other way as well.

Practise thought hygiene

With all the chatter going on in there, it's no wonder it gets a bit loud and confusing in our heads! Feed the good thoughts. Take leadership over your own thinking and train yourself to bring your thoughts into alignment with your vision. Do this consciously and daily. The minute you wake up, set your daily course.

Some of us spend too much of our lives in the metaphorical dining room of our minds and not enough in the other rooms living our life. Contrary to the way some of us act, we weren't born to think constantly about food and eat all day. Food, as we know, is for providing the fuel and nutrition that our physical bodies require, with the added bonus of the pleasure of sharing good food with families and friends. It should not only be good for the body, but good for the soul.

Those of you who work at home whether looking after family, earning a living, or retired know that the lure of the fridge can be a killer when it comes to trying to stay on the right path. It is always there enticing us with the thought of leftover dinners or puddings that need to be cleaned up (don't want to waste food) or snacks and treats that are hidden away in the pantry that keep calling out your name. Couple this with our tendency to look for the distraction of pleasure we are sure must be somewhere in the fridge when we are feeling varying degrees of pain, then the kitchen can physically be a trap.

Just like the physical issue of being surrounded by food, spending too much time in the kitchen of our minds can be a major hindrance to reaching our wellbeing goals. And we are not engaging in what life is really all about and therefore not living the lives we were meant to live. I know the food chatter in our heads can drive us crazy. I'm saying get out of the kitchen, move away from the fridge. Both literally and figuratively.

Find meaning and joy in all the other things that life is all about. Our work. Playing with our children and being present with them. Reading books and allowing our thoughts and imaginations to expand our world. Learning new things. Enjoying nature. Singing in the choir. Joining clubs or groups who do interesting things. All the things that engage the other parts of your human self and create a balanced, happy life.

If you are constantly thinking about food and what you should eat and whether you should eat and why you shouldn't eat, then you are missing out on life.

Emotional state

We can be as grown up as you like, fully functioning members of society, professionally respected etc. but in our emotional lives and in our weakest moments, we can sometimes be on par with a two-year-old toddler.

My weakest moments are those when I am tired or feel a bit down. The day has not gone right and I turn to food to change my state from that feeling to one of pleasure. Instant pleasure. We've all had experience of that child who when their will is thwarted and they can't get what they want, they throw a fit and cry and yell like it was the end of the world. No, you can't have those lollies because they will spoil the dinner of delicious nutritious foods prepared for you to make you strong and healthy, to help you grow into a well-balanced, resilient, healthy individual. BUT I WANT LOLLIES!!!!!.

One of the well-known building blocks to maturity is delayed gratification. Children who are developing normally will learn this and mature into successful adulthood. You are an adult and as a sign of maturity, you can relearn how to deal with those emotions. You have free will. The more you choose those new pathways that lead to your goals, the more you are likely to get there.

One of the main reasons we put on weight is not because we are eating normal meals but because of our indulgence in what is essentially children's party foods. What are children's party foods? Lollies, doughnuts, chocolate, chips, ice-cream. Foods that are great for special occasions but not great if you eat them too often. The experience of pleasure is fleeting and the consequences of this pattern of behaviour are part of our pain.

One of the characteristics of the inner child behaviour is not thinking at all but being fully involved in the emotion. As a child grows up, they will start to think about the adult's explanation of why they can't have lollies five minutes before dinner and work out the wisdom and logic of that. They will realise that is better for them as a whole person to eat well. And the more mature we get, the more we listen to that voice. Some of us need to be reminded of that.

If we carry on acting like a child and blindly trying to feed our emotions with treats in a vain attempt to move from pain to pleasure, we are continually feeding and rewarding that behaviour. Behaviour we reward and repeat builds habit. Remind yourself of how time works and how what you do today determines your future and make another choice.

 Do not be discouraged when you identify long held patterns and behaviours that are stopping you reaching your goals in any part of your life – not just health. You can overcome them through the process of first recognising and identifying them, and then replacing them with new helpful and whole practices.

Cultivate a mindset of success. Feed your soul.

The best way to find and keep the sort of mindset that creates the right environment for success is to feed your soul. Even Jesus Himself said, *"Man does not live by bread alone."* It is not just food we need to nourish our bodies; we need good positive useful input into our minds on a regular basis. If you have ever been on a personal growth course, read a good self-help book, or listened to an inspirational speaker and gone away feeling uplifted, then that is the state of mind I am talking about. Keep feeding that part of yourself to ensure you keep growing in personal strength.

Surround yourself with positive people who understand your journey. Have a friend or two and meet together to share your burdens and rejoice in your successes. I find I can easily get bogged down in what I perceive as a problem and a good friend may approach it with a fresh pair of eyes to point out the (sometimes obvious) solution. Maybe you can get a life coach - someone who has been here before you and helps show you the way.

Never in history have we had so many fantastic inspirational speakers available to us at any time of the day or night. Check out YouTube and find someone you can identify with. There are many inspirational books out there. One of the most important things you can do for yourself is to keep that input going. It will go a long way to helping you reach your goals.

A daily diet of soul food will be just as helpful to your success as eating the right kinds of food and taking the right kinds of exercise.

Success Work. How can I clean up my own physical environment to support my new goals. What strategies can I use to manage my internal thoughts to stop them going down the old negative pathways. How can I feed my soul? What other steps can I take to ensure my environment supports my new goal – not keep me at my old one.

Stage 5

Winning The Race

Success comes by putting what you have learned into practice: tailor it to fit your life.

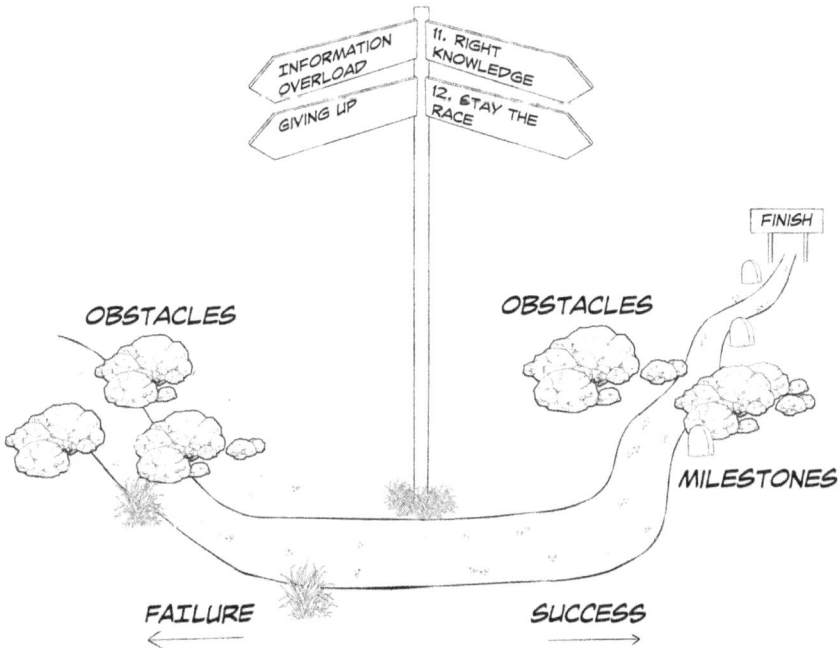

Chapter 11

The Right Knowledge

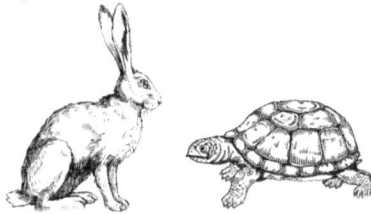

How often have we been stopped from doing something because we did not know what to do? Having the right knowledge and then applying it to your circumstances and lifestyle will go a long way to you reaching your own personal goals.

With all the information out there, it is hard to cut through and get to the heart of why we put on weight and what the best way is to lose it. I know my eyes have sometimes glazed over when another new piece of diet magic gets reported on in the media. Information, however, can become useful when it comes with context.

In this chapter we will take a quick look at some of key areas where the right knowledge will really help you understand why we need to eat the way we should, and not just because someone tells you to, but because it becomes deeply and life changingly relevant to you personally. Entire books have been written on these topics, so I am really giving you a summary of what works and you can look further into what you feel you need to do. In fact you will need to do some of your own research into what works for you at your stage in life.

Food as nutrition

Probably the biggest change in thinking that I came to understand when working on the *Tortoise Diet Method* was seeing food not just as calories, which tends to be the focus of traditional diets, or even as fellowship, but as nutrition. Once you understand why you need the nutrients that good whole food provides, you are better able to make those choices. And once you get into the habit of making those good choices part of your new normal in life, your increasingly glowing good health will make it much easier to live your best life, including getting your weight into balance.

We need the nutrients that food provides for energy of course, which is why we need calories, but also because they drive all the bodily functions required for life. I knew nothing of the role of hormones or the whole cascade of biochemical reactions necessary to life going on unseen within my body before learning this. The food we eat, the macronutrients of protein, fat and carbohydrate and the micronutrients of trace elements, vitamins and minerals are the source of what is needed to ensure all those systems get what they need in order to work properly.

This is why eating from a wide range of vegetables, fruits, nuts, and other whole foods is so important to our health and wellbeing. We need to ensure that we get what we need to be well. Most of us are just idling along because we overload our bodies with too much in the way of low nutrient-dense foods. The more you live this way and the older you get, the more likely your proverbial spark plugs are going to get blocked up or you could something really major is going to blow. Think how you would feel if you increased the nutrients - not only would you look fab, but you would feel fab as well!

So, what are these nutrients and how are they going to help me reach my goals?

Carbohydrates

It may surprise you to learn that fruits and vegetables are carbohydrates. I know I always used to associate carbs with starchy vegetables, bread, sugar, pasta, rice, wheat, and other grains. But anything that tastes sweet and contains sugars come under the category of carbohydrates.

Carbohydrates have had a lot of bad press lately, mainly because we now have a much greater understanding of why too much sugar in our system is so dangerous to our health. We also have more knowledge of the hormonal response our body has to sugar and that has led to some people cutting out all carbohydrates as a food group.

It's become a much more prevalent issue in the past few decades because of the massive increase in sugar in the modern diet. Sugar in various forms is being added to just about every form of processed food out there. When the prevalent diet thinking of a few years ago was that fat was the enemy, fat was taken out of food and replaced with sugar and salt. As a result of that, we are eating way more sugar and salt than ever before, whether we know it or not.

What we now know is that when we eat carbohydrate, it is broken down in our bodies into sugar as glucose and enters our bloodstream. It can't stay there as it's harmful to the blood vessels so to get it out of there, the hormone insulin is released from our pancreas into the blood and it then accompanies the unwanted sugar off to our muscles and liver where it is turned into glycogen and used by the body when it needs quick access to readily available energy. So far, so good.

Normally (and by normally I mean for most of human history when we didn't have access to the carbohydrates we now have in abundance) the occasional and seasonal increase in insulin in our system was balanced out by the production of another hormone called leptin. Leptin is the satiety hormone which kicks in when we've eaten enough. In this case 'enough' is indicated by the high level of insulin in the system, which in turn is generated by the high level of sugar in the system.

However, recent studies have shown that if the insulin is too high, then the ability of the brain to detect leptin is reduced. So, you now have the ironic situation that your insulin level has to come down before the leptin can do its proper work. Can you see how our modern eating patterns are making it so hard for us?

Nowadays, with the endless forms of sweet sugary treats available at all times of the day the many spikes in our blood sugar levels require more and more insulin being secreted in order to take care of it. We now have too much sugar in our systems and our muscles and liver no longer have the capacity to store it. So, what happens instead? Insulin then moves it for storage into that space of potentially endless capacity - our fat cells. Insulin is the fat storage hormone, ladies and gentlemen, and we keep asking our pancreas to pump it into our blood when we eat sugar. We can try all we like to release weight, but if we keep overloading our bodies with regular supplies of sugar, then we are making it very hard to do so. The constant pumping of insulin into our bloodstream to counteract the constant pumping of sugar into our blood stream has led to a prevalence of insulin resistance – a precursor to type 2 diabetes.

But don't just suddenly cut out all forms of carbohydrate from your diet like the hare would do. Our bodies need glucose in the system to power the brain and provide quick burning energy throughout the day, so we need to eat the right carbohydrates. We get a lot of our nutrition from these plant foods – we just need to eat them in the right forms and the right proportions to meet our specific needs. They provide us with the dietary fibre needed for good gut health, promote elimination, slow down the absorption of the sugars into our bloodstream and help to fill us up. Plants contain antioxidants that are essential to the maintenance of our immune system and help us fight disease.

If we choose carefully, we can provide for our nutritional needs and help with weight loss rather than contribute to it. For instance, most leafy green vegetables, fruits, and wholegrains come pre-packaged with lots of dietary fibre. The good news is that because this fibre slows down the entry of the sugars into the bloodstream, and therefore the amount of insulin entering, there is less spiking either in the way of blood sugar being dumped or massive doses of insulin produced.

Surprisingly, one of the most harmful sugars is that found in fruit known as fructose. Unfortunately, it shows up as an almost universal component of processed food (corn syrup) in our modern system disguised as being good for you. Avoid it where it shows up in processed foods but eating fruit in moderation with all the attendant vitamins, minerals and fibre means the good far outweighs the bad. Moderation means no more than a couple of pieces of fruit per day.

The other good news is to eat some good protein at every meal because the hormone glucagon, released when we eat protein, does the opposite of insulin and encourages fat burning.

The Tortoise Diet Method is about a moderate use of carbohydrates in the diet rather than cutting them all out. I don't cut out bread altogether, for instance, but I do choose really good bread when I have it. As I listened to my body more, I noticed that my tolerance for bread and wheat products was reducing. Some of them started to give me a feeling of indigestion after I ate them and so I am naturally choosing to eat less.

Interestingly, some studies show that women rather than men store carbs as fat and menopausal women do it even more so. As a menopausal woman, listening to my body when it is telling me to eat less starchy processed carbs such as some breads is making sense. This is a good example of adapting what you eat to what works for you at your stage in life.

There is another sneaky little problem with sugar that can affect your attempts at losing weight. One reason for the way our body reacts to sugar by pressing the 'store' button is that it could have something to do with the way we were designed. Normally in nature, sweet foods are available from late summer into autumn, just in time for us to want to be putting on some extra weight to carry us through the scarcity of winter.

It seems that in order to encourage the eating of these sweeties, their consumption caused the pleasure area of our brain to spark up so that we would naturally want to repeat the behaviour. Experiments have shown that the feel-good hormone, dopamine, shows up in our brain even when we just look at something sweet, let alone eat it. That's our limbic subconscious system kicking in again, pushing us into the behaviour it thinks we need to survive. Trouble is back then; sweet things were scarce. No need to point out that now we are bombarded with not just way too much sugar but images as well, setting us up to get our next dopamine fix. No wonder it's a hard habit to break.

Because the *Tortoise Diet Method* is concerned with sustainability, I am hesitant to say cut out all the carbs that we associate with a normal nutritious family meal, like rice, pasta or potato, for example. I would suggest, however, that you reduce the portion-size of them and increase the amount of coloured leafy vegetables. Even better if you choose brown rice or wholewheat pasta.

From that point, as you get more comfortable and accustomed to the idea, swap them out for zucchini noodles, or cruciferous vegetables such as cauliflower or broccoli. If I am making a winter casserole, for instance, I don't even miss not having a starchy carb such as potato or rice with it if I just serve it on a bed of steamed vegetables. It's just as delicious and gets me to my goal quicker. Listen to your body, try new things, and let the results guide you.

We all need to cut back as much as we can on our sugar consumption wherever it is. The WHO recommends no more than twelve teaspoons of sugar per day, but a lot of other agencies are recommending even less. A teaspoon of sugar is 4g, so when you look at the nutrition guide on a product, divide the total sugars by 4 to get the number of teaspoons. You'll probably get a real shock about the amount hidden in your diet.

Other ways you can cut down is by cutting out any fizzy drinks or sodas, encourage your kids to drink water, eat your fruit rather than drink fruit juice, stop buying and eating processed muesli bars, cookies, confectionery and so on. You will feel better, look better and your Dentist will be happier as well.

Since we need all the goodness provided by the good plant foods, how can we avoid this over-abundance of insulin and the ensuing fat storage issue? Let's look at the next important food macronutrient that you need: Protein.

Protein

Protein provides the ingredients for all the amino acids in your body vital to making us function properly, so it is your friend when it comes to eating right for your health. We need protein because it provides the basis for amino acids. We need those because they create and support our immune system and the neurotransmitters in our brain. Protein is also a key component of maintaining and building your muscle mass – vitally important if you want to burn excess fat. So quite important then.

When we eat protein, another hormone known as glucagon is released that tells your body to move fat into your bloodstream and use it as energy. Not store it like insulin does. Eating protein along with carbohydrates helps to maintain the right level of sugars in your blood.

Fat

Before we came back to the knowledge that it is more likely that too much sugar in the system is the primary culprit for our inability to lose weight, fat was the bogeyman. For a while, food that was promoted as fat free was all the rage. The trouble was fat is a flavour carrier. You remove the fat from food, and it turns into a tasteless time-waster. To make up for this lack, more sugar and salt was added plus various other artificial chemical concoctions to make the processed product palatable. It also meant that it ended up far worse for you than if it just had the original fat left in it. A generation of overweight people can testify to that.

Fats are not only flavour carriers, but they help to satisfy us. When we go back to eating whole foods containing friendly fats we find our natural appetites again. It only takes a small amount of fat to make us feel full and so it is quite hard to overeat the natural fats we find in plants, dairy, and meat. The same cannot be said for the hidden and altered fats found in over processed foods. Commercial biscuits, pastries, ice-cream, confectionary, sauces and so on are all likely to have some kind of trans or altered fats and sugars added. In the interests of profit margins, food manufacturers are more likely to use cheap oils and fats in their food production. What we may save in money will end up eventually costing us far more in health.

Be careful of the fats that come in the form of oils as well. Many can lead to a high level of inflammation in the body. Good fats such as those found in avocado, olives, flaxseed and oily fish reduce inflammation, contribute to the health of your joints, skin, eyes and brain, help to lower cholesterol in the blood and also help keep weight down because our hunger is satisfied by the consumption of it.

Vitamins and minerals
Sometimes referred to as trace elements, vitamins and minerals are needed In tiny regular amounts, which is why they are called 'trace' elements. Vitamins are a vital part of our biochemistry and needed to provide the information to build and maintain our body, support our immune system, and fight disease.

Minerals is a term you may have heard of but have had little understanding of where they fit in. Minerals themselves form the actual building material of our bodies: our bones, for example, our teeth – even our cartilage. There are certain minerals we need daily to stay strong and healthy. A shortlist of these would include: iron, calcium, copper, magnesium, phosphorus, potassium, selenium, and zinc.

You can get them from supplements, but the best way is from your food. Science has not yet reproduced the whole benefits that come from eating a head of broccoli, for instance. This is a good example of the whole not being the sum of its parts. As the French would say, there is an element of the *je ne sai quoi* in the whole food, especially naturally grown in well-nourished soil and grown close to home, that you cannot yet get out of a bottle. Eating a wide range of foods is the best way to get these into your body in the right form.

Vitamins and minerals come from eating leafy green vegetables, fruits, eggs, protein, wholegrains, pulses, dairy food, yoghurt, meats, fish, shellfish, nuts, and seeds.

Whole foods

Our bodies know what food is because we have adapted over time to the food available to us. What happens if you take a component out of the whole food and then ask the body to use and absorb this new thing? Even worse, what if you genetically modify what used to be food and present that as food? At some level, our bodies do not recognise it and do what needs to be done in order to protect itself from this unknown organism. Inflammation, auto-immune responses, and ultimately one form of ill health or another can result in response to a diet high in processed or altered foods. Choose food as much as you can as close as you can to its original source if you want the best health.

Processed foods

A study reported in the Georgia State University News in February 2015 reported on an experiment where mice were fed two emulsifying agents commonly added to foods. The animals in the study gained weight, had altered blood sugar, and developed intestinal problems. What these emulsifiers did that changed food from its natural state was to hold together fat and water that would normally be separate in real food. In this case, both inflammation and metabolic syndrome was triggered in the mice. This is one study and, of course, they concluded that more study needed to be done to determine the effect on humans, but it is one of the clues we need to point us away from commercially processed food in our diets.

One good definition of a processed food is one that looks nothing like its original form. Biscuits look nothing like wheat, for instance, but a chop looks like a chop when it is cooked and served on a plate. Much of the wheat used today to make all of our biscuits and breads and pastries looks nothing like the original wheat used even 100 years ago. It has been modified to help with rate of production, but this has come at a cost to nutrition. People who have allergies to modern wheat often find they don't have the same response to earlier forms of wheat or more ancient grains.

Ironically, when sugar from sugar cane first made it to the Old World a few hundred years ago, it was so rare and such a status symbol that only the rich ate it. As a result, there was a lot of aristocratic rotting of the teeth going on, Queen Elizabeth I included. It was the poor who had the good teeth. These days, it's the other way round. It's the poor that are more likely to choose cheap processed sugar-laden products that result in poor dental health now. Same goes for white flour. When the process to strip flour of its germ and bran was industrialised and white bread became fashionable amongst the wealthy, no cucumber sandwich could ever be thinner or whiter. Now again, it's more likely to be the poor who eat the white commercial bread and those who can afford it choosing the lovely artisanal wholegrain breads.

Gut health

An important part of the well-being story is gut health. You will hear more and more about the importance of gut health as scientists are rediscovering earlier knowledge about the role this plays in our lives.

In terms of the physical component, we know that we each have a unique population of gut bacteria known as microbiome located in our digestive system. It can weigh up to 3 kilos and that is 3 kilos you don't want to lose! We are coming to understand more and more about the importance of those bacteria to our health and wellbeing – and weight loss.

A good healthy microbiome is going to better be able to digest the food going in. They seem to produce the right enzymes to break down starch into the smaller components needed for our body to use to function. If that can be done efficiently and we are getting what we need, then the body doesn't need to send those emergency messages to us to say, "I haven't got enough food to keep you going, so eat more!"

There are many more ways good gut health contributes to our wellbeing. It can protect us from illnesses. As I write these chapters, we are hearing a lot about viruses. We need to get the message out there that increasing our gut health is the first step in protecting ourselves and our families from such attacks. The microbes in our gut can go into action, prevent the virus from growing and neutralise toxins produced by the virus. Healthy microbes can boost our immune system by strengthening the white blood cells that are the key player in our defence against foreign invaders such as viruses, bacteria, or parasites.

Good bacteria can crowd out bad bacteria as well. Making the gut environment more suitable for the good will make it less welcoming to the bad ones. They can do this by making lactic acid and fatty acids which lower the pH inside the colon, which is less attractive to the bad ones.

Which brings me back to what to eat. We can't get away from the message that eating foods not only rich in fibre but rich in different types of fibre are all going to be helpful to maintaining a good environment for these little guys. It also takes me back to traditional ways of eating. Most cultures have a fermented food in their diet - yoghurt, pickled vegetables such as kimchi or sauerkraut. All great for supporting good gut health.

The good news is that we can maintain the right conditions for the beneficial ones to thrive, and in doing so, we are more likely to thrive. This gives us another reason to eat from a wide range of foods as we work to encourage a wide range of different types of bacteria.

The importance of protecting and increasing our gut biome extends to what not to eat. In the past few decades, a lot of attention, corporate energy, and resources have gone into messing around with real food. Adding this, subtracting that, substituting and synthesising, and it is highly likely that we are seeing the results in the increase in food allergies, immune response and weight gain. Our bodies and gut simply do not recognise the altered foods we feed them. This is why you need to avoid over processed foods as much as you can.

Fibre

I am sure you are starting to understand the importance of dietary fibre in your diet as you read this chapter. Because fibre is bulky it can fill up your stomach which then causes the release of the hormone cholecystokinin (CKK). This then signals to the brain that you are full and therefore slow down with the appetite signals.

It takes longer for the body to process fibre, which is why it slows down entry of sugar into the bloodstream and reduces the incidence of insulin spiking. It also takes more energy for the body to burn while processing than other foods – so adding plenty of fibre to the diet will help burn more calories.

As with all changes you make to your body, do not suddenly add a lot of fibre to your diet. Keep coming back to the tortoise and take it slowly at first until your gut has adjusted. Drink plenty of water while you are doing that. Just remember that any changes to your diet will also affect your gut flora, whether they are good changes or bad. The principle of feeding the good and starving the bad, whether it is for our gut, or our thoughts or behaviours, is the best way to make the necessary changes that will last.

Water

You hear a lot in weight-loss circles about the importance of drinking water. It is not always easy to make that change and it can just seem pointless (apart from all the exercise you may get from going to the bathroom so often) so why all the water?

Water can help your body use up stored fat. The liver is the biggest organ involved in weight loss. One of its primary functions is to turn fat into fuel for the body. If you don't drink enough water, your kidneys, which also act as filters, don't have enough fluid to flush what it needs to out of your body, so the liver has to join in to help. If it is doing that, it can't do its proper job of metabolizing fat and so your fat loss slows down. This is a good example of knowledge driving behaviour. Once I learned this, it became a lot easier to down that water!

It is not just its role in metabolizing fat, either. Drinking plenty of water during the day can reduce hunger by keeping our stomachs full. Water flushes out the waste products released as our digestion is activated and, of course, we look a lot better when we are nicely hydrated!

It is best not to drink water for thirty minutes either side of eating a meal or with a meal. The reason is to do with digestion and the stomach acid we need to properly process our food. Good health is linked to good digestion and water can dilute your stomach acid so increase your intake outside of mealtimes.

Liver health

I know I have said that the brain might be the biggest fat burning organ in the body, but I was possibly being a bit facetious there because it can be more about the way we think than the way we eat. However, I know that the liver is equally up there. We lose weight best when our bodies are operating like they were meant to and it is very hard to do that unless we look after our liver. So, if you think you are doing all you can in terms of calorie restriction to lose weight, but nothing much is working for you, then paying attention to your liver might help.

The liver helps with weight loss because it turns all the problematic substances we eat (or enter through our skin or respiratory system) into a form that is less dangerous for our body and then eliminates it through excretion. This includes excess fat. There are two reasons it can't always do this job properly.

One is that there are not enough nutrients in your food to make the enzymes needed to do the work. The other is that we overload the liver with too many things that need to be taken care of. We overeat, or we eat all the time, and as a result the liver never gets a break or a chance to catch up. This is another reason that the foods we eat that either contribute to our health and wellbeing are the same ones that will support good weight loss. Too much alcohol, too much caffeine, too much sugar, especially those industrial grade ones, the wrong kinds of fat plus all the chemicals in the environment found in skincare, beauty products, pesticides, building material or drugs. This just sounds like the modern way of life, really.

But foods that contain Vitamin B, antioxidants, amino acids, sulphur, and selenium are all going to be helpful. This includes whole grains, eggs, onion and garlic, cabbage, cauliflower, broccoli, and kale. There is some good herbal support out there for the liver, and this may be something that you would find helpful. Spend some time doing your own research into the importance of the liver and what applies to you.

Sleep
You've probably heard the phrase about getting your beauty sleep. Getting enough sleep contributes to well-being, looking good and weight loss alike. If you don't get enough sleep and you are tired and grumpy, you can produce the hormone cortisol, which breaks down the collagen in our skin and highlights our wrinkles!

If that's not bad enough, lack of sleep can interfere with the production of our appetite control hormones with the result that the one that reminds us to eat (ghrelin) wins out over the one that says to stop eating (leptin). That old stress hormone, cortisol, can also increase, messing around with our insulin and stopping us from burning fat. It just seems to make sense that if you are tired and grumpy and sleep deficient, you have less resistance to overeating sweet treats as well. Just make sure you get enough sleep!

The importance of including protein in your evening meal is highlighted when you realise that protein produces the amino acid tryptophan, which is a precursor to the sleep hormone, melatonin. Eating good quality protein at each meal is going to contribute to a good night's sleep. On the other hand, too much sugar in your system delays the release of melatonin and can interfere with sleep.

Being overweight means that you carry extra fat around the neck as well – this can lead to snoring but also to the sleep disorder known as Sleep Apnoea. Even losing 5-10% of your body weight will help with getting a better night's sleep and continue to help with weight loss.

Alcohol

As always, take a moderate approach to alcohol if you can't cut it out altogether. It's unnecessary in any nutritional sense, but it can be part of our enjoyment of food and life in our culture. It can be full of sugar, and it is a liver loader, so you will get better results the more you reduce it. It also reduces inhibitions, and you will end up eating way more if you drink too much. I'm a bit of a one glass wonder, so if I drink any more than that, I have to say goodbye to any sensible food restraint. Try finding some good non-alcoholic replacements that you will enjoy. If you do choose to drink alcohol, make sure you choose something that is really good quality, drink it in moderation and jolly well enjoy it! The pain/pleasure continuum applies here.

Exercise

Just as when it comes to the approach to diets, one size of exercise does not fit all. However, no matter what age or stage you are, there are some things you need to do for your wellbeing and weightloss success. One is to just move. Sometimes difficult when you spend a lot of your day sitting on your bottom in front of a computer screen but find a way to move during the course of your day.

Walking is my favourite and can be done by most people at most stages of life. Walking helps the body maintain health by keeping all your body processes moving, including your lymph glands, and also burns energy. It is a form of cardio-vascular exercise which, while it has a lot of health benefits, is less useful directly to fat loss than the next form of exercise.

The other is to do some kind of muscle building exercise. Your metabolic rate is directly linked to your muscle mass so making some effort towards growing and maintaining your muscle is a very important part of losing and keeping weight off.

Your basic metabolic rate is the amount of energy required to keep all your systems maintained and your body working in order to keep you alive. That goes for all the automatic processes that are constantly taking place, such as breathing, digestion, maintaining body temperature, and keeping your organs functioning. Lean body tissue (muscle) uses up more energy than plain old fat in this equation so the more muscle you have, the more your body will burn up calories even while you sleep!

Building muscle comes about by resistance training or strength training. This could be lifting weights, gardening (getting up and down is resistance training) stretching or movement exercises such as Pilates. This does not mean you have to turn into a gym bunny - in fact, you still need to be a gym tortoise when it comes to behaviour around that. Regularly repeating the right exercises in small doses over time is always better than going to the gym for a few weeks, overdoing it, then giving up. If the gym environment suits you and your lifestyle then take advantage of the knowledge provided by the trainers and work out what specific exercises you can do to increase muscle mass.

Muscle mass naturally reduces as we get older or stop using them as much. The longer you can maintain or even build muscle mass, the more you will burn fat and keep a healthy weight. There are some I work on because I want to look better. Flabby arms where the fat continues to wave long after I have finished waving goodbye to visitors, or a wobbly belly. Working on your core (which includes that wobbly belly) not only makes you look better, but holds all your important organs in the right places.

As with everything in the *Tortoise Diet Method*, find out what works for you and do that.

Intermittent fasting and time restricted eating

Once you have cleared yourself of those old patterns and are a good way down the path of practising the right steps to reach your goal, there is no reason you can't do a bit extra toward your end result.

All science should be moving forward and updating itself as new information becomes available, including nutritional science. One example is the new knowledge about something called intermittent fasting. Studies have suggested (most notably from Professor Roy Taylor's work published in 2018) that there are benefits from losing weight rapidly in a short period of time. Now this is where us old yoyo dieters must be careful, because that has been pretty much what we tried and failed to do for most of our adult lives. We have been more about intermittent weight gain than anything else! So, what is intermittent fasting all about?

Fasting can be a real trigger word – its success really depends on the reason why you are doing it and what sort of fasting you are doing. Fasting can mean abstaining from food for a period until a certain prearranged result has been achieved. This is often a spiritual practice and has nothing to do with losing weight. Abstaining from eating *in order to lose weight* will never work for most of us, for all the reasons we have already covered in this book; our metabolism just shuts down to protect life and compels us to find food to eat in order to survive. It just messes with our bodies and our minds.

A specific form of fasting with the deliberate aim of losing weight quickly over a short period of time has recently been popularised in the books by Dr Michael Mosley and his *Fast 800* Diet method. There are two ways you can do this and safely incorporate it into your *Tortoise Diet Method.* One is that you eat moderately for 5 days a week (just like I would recommend anyway) within a certain window of time, but the other 2 days you do a partial fast of consuming only 800 calories per day. This is called the 5:2 method. I have tried this but still found the restriction on the 2 days triggered my old unhelpful "diet" mentality and behavioural patterns that I want to avoid.

The other way is something that is helpful and that is why I recommend under Guidepost 2 that you stop eating after 7pm and have breakfast a bit later in the morning. This is called *Time Restricted Eating*, where you eat your meals within a specified window of time during the day, leaving a good long gap where nothing is eaten. Divide your day into 24 hours and only eat within a window between 12 to 8 hours of them – starting with what you can manage first.

Again, you must watch your propensity to take anything to extremes and impose unnecessary rules on yourself, but you can safely eat within a window of between 8 to 12 hours a day in line with the

Tortoise Diet Method and still get good results over time. This just means having your breakfast say between 9am or 10am and evening meal by 6.00pm.

It can work well, especially as hunger is rarely an issue first thing in the morning. It is easy to delay breakfast. It might even be more practical if you are a commuter and need to leave the house very early in the morning. Eating your breakfast at the traditional morning tea time of 10am would work well. Then three hours later have lunch. Have your afternoon snack if you can't safely wait until your evening meal, but if you can, have an early dinner. Then get into the habit of not eating after dinner.

There are some good reasons the practise of time restricted eating and intermittent fasting works and may be helpful to you along the way. Both practises talk about something called autophagy. The word itself means to 'self-eat' and works by repairing the body – literally eating up old dead damaged cells and then create new ones. It can only do this when you are not eating and then stops when you eat again. It is triggered after a period of a few hours of fasting. Is there not a better reason to hold fire on the evening snacks?

Your body will normally take around 6-8 hours after a meal to switch from burning glycogen to burning fat and it burns it even faster after you have not eaten for twelve hours. I aim to go sixteen hours and then eat within an eight-hour window for at least for 5 days a week. Usually those days during the week when I am focused on working. But I didn't jump straight into that pattern. I started with just stopping eating after dinner and then pushing my breakfast time back a bit. This is not hard and may help you greatly with sustaining good, steady weight loss without too much effort. This may be something that you can start to make into a habit of your own.

What to eat

You may have noticed that there are no recipes in this book. The reason for that is because if you take a quick look around your kitchen I am guessing you will see plenty of cookbooks full of recipes, most of which you probably haven't tried. The whole point of the *Tortoise Diet Method* is that you eat as normally as you can while making the adjustments suggested above. That way you are more likely to sustain a lifelong heathy way of eating.

You also need to find what suits you and your way of life, your food preferences and particular health conditions. This book would be very long if we covered off all the possible dietary requirements and life stages out there, plus I am not pushing a particular diet but a whole way of eating for health and wellbeing. Become your own expert for what you need to eat and make what works a regular part of your daily life.

I will put some suggestions on my social media platforms from time to time so keep checking in there if you wish but why not write your own personal diet book? Start collecting your own recipes that work for you and your family. Explore all those recipe books on your shelf and adapt some to suit.

Like a lot of things with the *Tortoise Diet Method*, there is a bit of a continuum with what to eat. There are some things that are enjoyable and make life liveable that are not necessarily the best thing to eat all the time but no one is going to eat the perfect diet all the time. What will work best is when we eat mostly what is good for our wellbeing most of the time.

The below table goes from what to avoid where you can, what to eat the most of when possible, and all the variations in between.

When I started on this *Method,* I ate mostly in the eat moderately column and as time went by moved more towards the eat mostly column. The further to the right of that continuum you eat the most of, the better your results so it is up to you where you choose to live most of the time.

I do want to put in a disclaimer here. I know that food and nutrition are just about as controversial now as politics and religion. This list is something that I have come up with based on reading the research of others and it is neither complete nor set in stone. It is not meant to be the bible – it is a guideline and a starting point. If you are vegan or vegetarian for example, your list will look different but will use the same principles. Some foods represent food categories, such as complex carbohydrates, and I don't have room to list them all. If you have other information and think that something else suits you better than by all means make some adjustments to suit you. There is a table for you to design for yourself in your workbook.

The Tortoise Diet Method Food Continuum

Move as much as you can from the left side of the table to the right side.

Avoid where possible	Eat less of	Consume Moderately	Eat mostly
Processed food. Artificially sweetened anything. Corn Syrup in anything. Fruit Juice. Trans fats. Highly processed vegetable oils like canola, rice bran, sunflower, corn, grapeseed and soyabean.	Carbs- white bread, white rice, white pasta, instant oats, processed breakfast cereals, Biscuits, cake and other high carb snack food, Chips Alcohol	Proteins: Processed meats like bacon, sausage, salami etc Carbs: Root vegetables, rice, whole pasta, bread, fruit Fats; Sesame Oil, Peanut Oil, Hemp Oil Alcohol	Proteins – oily fish, fish, seafood, chicken, meat, eggs, tofu, beans, pulses, cheese, yoghurt, nuts and seeds. Carbs – Green and coloured leafy vegetables, incl. brassicas, onions, garlic and other non starchy vegetables. Complex carbs rich in fibre. Good fats; Eg avocado, olive, macadamia or nut oils, fish oils, Flaxseed oils, Butter

Success Work. Apply this knowledge to your situation and come up with your own solution. Come up with your own meal plans. Write your own recipe book to include meals you enjoy that work for you and your family. Apply the Food Continuum Table to you. What will you eat most of to get the best results.

Chapter 12

YOUR Strategy for Success

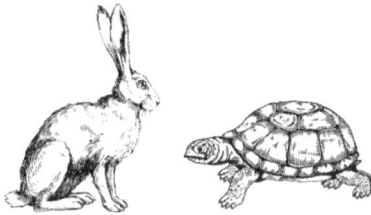

Now comes the time to put this all into practise. We can't just keep learning without living out what we learn if we really want to be effective. The final piece needed is to make this whole process into your own personal roadmap towards your own goals. One that is tailored to your time of life, circumstances, age or stage, whatever that might be. Come up with your own strategy to deal with the problems you can now recognise as they raise their heads. Take the leadership in your own life and get excited about the fact that you are the boss of you, and you can have a hand in creating your own future!

We've had some fun with the ancient fable, taking the metaphor from it of your weight loss journey being like a race and learning from the behaviour of each of the characters within what to do more of and what to stop doing. This race is less like a sprint than a marathon, so I have structured it to match the stages you will typically go through when you plan on winning.

I have divided the successful race up into five stages.
- Losing the race – where we have spent much of our lives.
- Getting the right strategy – dropping what hasn't worked and do what does.
- The starting line – getting equipped and getting the right finish line in sight.
- Running the race – putting the right behaviour into practise over time.
- Winning the race – living according to the vision of your best self.

Within each of these stages are the guideposts to show you the way to go. If you follow these and make them part of your life then they will show you how to win. Then there are milestones along the way – ones you will be able to create for yourself to represent reaching those goals you have not been able to achieve for a long time. The following is a summary of those steps found in the *Tortoise Diet Method* that when you apply to your own life you will go a long way to winning that race after all.

Stage 1. Losing the Race

Guidepost 1. Stop Dieting
The first two Chapters of the book help you start to understand where you were at the beginning of your journey. Answer the

questions and do your own audit of your life, then make the connection between what is going on in your life and your weight journey. Start to work out why traditional diets have not worked for you and the reasons why you have put on weight. Most importantly of all Guidepost 1 calls you to stop the old dieting behaviour and start to let go of all that terrible pressure you have put on yourself in the past, walk away from the old, disordered thinking and behaviour and start considering a new approach.

Part of that audit is to take a physical benchmark of where you are now so you will know how far you have come as you start to hit those goals. Make a record of your vital statistics such as your weight and your measurements. It might be interesting to note down where you feel you are in terms of your mental and emotional health as well.

Stage 2. The Right Strategy

Any athlete who wants to win a race must have the right strategy – which is what the *The Tortoise Diet Method* really is. It looks at the individual approaches of the hare and the tortoise and observes what you can learn about your own behaviour. That includes what it takes to lose and what it takes to win. You will find the right strategy in Chapters two, three, four and five.

Guidepost 2. Reset your eating

Under the Chapter heading "The Great Reset" the action for this guidepost is to get into the habit of eating 3 normal moderate nutritious meals a day. Make sure they are not too far from your normal to start with. Get inspiration from what you grew up with, what is ancestral (part of your family culture and tradition) what is seasonal and what you and your family like.

Plan them carefully to include plenty of protein, good fats and the right carbohydrates to create a healthy body. Start where you are and then gradually add more vegetables, and cut back on unnecessary carbohydrates, especially sugar. Stop eating processed and altered foods wherever you can. Repeat what works.

Make sure those meals are nutritious and they give the body what it needs to reduce the need for snacking in between. It's usually what you eat between meals that has the empty calories and is the main cause of weight gain. The exceptions are to eat a good protein based snack in the afternoon if there is too much of a gap between lunch and dinner, and to enjoy a little of what your fancy when joining in with celebrations- this is what life is all about.

The aim of this guidepost is to reset what is normal for you by starting where you are right now and slowly making the changes over time until eating what works for you becomes your new normal. What works for you is the food that keeps you strong, healthy and your weight at the right balance. Guidepost 2 can be found in Chapter 4.

Guidepost 3. Set an achievable goal

Under the Chapter 5 heading, *Wait Not Weight*, the action for this guidepost is to aim to lose 1 kilo a month over the course of a year. This may have been a bit hard to get your head around at first as we have always been told to set high goals with the thinking behind that being that we will stretch ourselves to meet them. However, in real life that has ended up setting most of us up for failure. I know it may seem counter intuitive but in this *Method* you start off with the very achievable goal of 1 kilo (about 2.2 pounds) a month – which anyone can do. Like the tortoise, break your journey down into small achievable steps. You will help to set yourself up for success as you start a new pattern of reaching those goals. It is far better to build slowly and spend time laying a good foundation for life-long success than to keep up a pattern of failing all the time.

It's what you do daily that counts so put the effort into doing what works each day and allowing the results to accumulate over time rather than expect quick results.

Guidepost 4. Measure wisely

In Chapter 6, *Stop Weighing Your Self-Esteem*, your action is to stop weighing yourself all the time and being emotionally tied into whatever that figure is. It urges you to take your focus off the weight and onto living in the right way to make losing weight and then keeping it off part of a normal healthy lifestyle. We are after a downward trend in your weight tracking over time. Stop the crazy daily weigh in – our bodies go up and down all the time when it comes to our weight and we tie far too much of our self-esteem up in what those scales say. Find other ways to measure your results – including your feeling of well-being!

However, the scales are useful as a benchmark to help measure your success so make your official weigh in once a month. Whatever you lose in the month, that new figure you reach becomes your starting point for the following month. Follow the buddy system if that helps with the psychology around this. Deal with any failure by learning from it and making sure you don't repeat what it was that led you there. Stop your pattern of escalating any small weight gain into a drama that stops you in your tracks.

Guidepost 5. The right exercise

Do the right exercise regularly that works for you at your stage in life. Focus on moving more throughout the day, stretching, and very importantly, increasing muscle mass by resistance training at least a couple of times a week so your muscles will burn energy even when you are asleep. You might even like to target an area of your body and learn exactly what exercise you need to tighten it up then repeat that every day. This is as opposed to going to the gym and doing a whole lot of exercises not very well and then giving up altogether.

Guidepost 4 can be found as part of the approach over time in Chapter 5 and as part of the right knowledge in Chapter 11.

Stage 3. The Starting Line

In stage 3 which is covered in Chapter 7 and 8, you are at the starting line. There are 2 important things here. You need to know where you are going, and you need to be properly equipped.

Guidepost 6. The Right Mindset

A few key mindset shifts at this stage will be a big help as you approach the race ahead of you. Understanding how time works – how the decisions you made in the past have affected where you are today and then how you can change your future by changing what you do today. Your future can also help you decide what actions you take today as we reverse engineer our compelling vision for our lives and do what we know will make that happen.

Having a healthy sense of self-worth, a good understanding of how you can have a hand in creating your own life once you understand you do have that power, plus taking on the attitude of a problem solver, will all be very helpful in the year ahead.

Guidepost 7. The Right Goal

Make sure you have the right goal – the clue is that it is not just a figure on the scales! A clear and compelling vision for your life - one that excites you and pulls you towards it will become your compass. Commit to it daily. Feel it with your emotions and visualise yourself already there. Use the power of visualisation, repetition, journalling, affirmation and intention in the context of all the positive emotion you can muster to anchor this goal in your soul.

Have a morning routine and take time to set yourself up for the day and care for yourself. Take leadership over your life, your thoughts, your behaviour, choose your emotional state, plan your day and plan your meals. Your motivation does not come from the sheer grunt of will power but comes from the power having a truly inspiring and compelling vision has in your life. Success will follow when you make a daily habit of commitment to that goal. Imagine yourself already that person and then do what you know that person would do in each situation you are confronted with.

Stage 4. Running the Race

Guidepost 8. The right thinking
You will find the value of having the right thoughts and beliefs in Chapter 9, *What Lies Beneath*. It will begin to help you understand why we seem so intent on sabotaging our own behaviour – even when we are trying to do what's right for us.

If our thoughts led us to where we are today, then they can also take us to where we want to go in the future. It's just that we have not necessarily been aware of what those thoughts have been. Our subconscious has a lot to say in the invisible programs we run beneath our consciousness. Depending on how powerful your hidden beliefs are and the effect they have on your life, this is one area that you may need to get some outside professional help with to help you uncover what lies beneath for you.

Guidepost 9. The right action

Chapter 9 also looks at how our actions reflect those inner beliefs and are a clue to uncovering unhelpful old patterns of behaviour. It will give you an insight into making the invisible visible and then what to do to replace those thoughts and beliefs. You can then start taking the right actions to getting the result you want. The power of habit forming is a key in this guidepost.

Guidepost 10. The right environment

Chapter 10, *Be the Boss of Your Environment* points to the very important role our internal and external environment has in both our failure and our success. Take the steps you need to in your environment to set it up to support your new direction and not keep going back to your old comfort zone. Create a new comfort zone that makes it easier to support your new behaviour.

Stage 5. Winning the Race

Winning the race comes down to tailoring this to fit your life and coming up with your own strategy.

Guidepost 11. The right knowledge

A guide to knowing where to look for the right knowledge can be found in Chapter 11. Although we can be overwhelmed with the amount of information we seem to be bombarded with, this gives you a starting point to then tailor it to your age and stage in life. One of the reasons diets have failed in the past is because they take a 'one size fits all' approach which doesn't work because we're not all the same size, shape, weight, age or stage. So find the right knowledge that applies to you.

Guidepost 12. Stay the Race

The final step is about sustainability – one of the keys lacking in traditional diet behaviour where we might lose weight but put it all back on once we finish the actual diet. Working your way through each step on the *Tortoise Diet Method* should address a lot of those issues. Adding in a determination to stick to it and follow through will mean you will win this time.

Obstacles: a new approach

With all of this in mind, revisit the list of obstacles you made earlier. Go through the exercise of looking at each one, note down what the *Tortoise Diet Method* approach would be, then note down what your strategic approach might be. There are a couple of examples below and more in your workbook.

Obstacle 1. Getting sick 2 weeks into a diet

TDM Solution. One reason this happens it that our subconscious doesn't like too much change so will resist and things come up for you – either in your body or in the world to stop you. Eating three nutritious meals a day that are not too far from normal with plenty of good food will ensure your subconscious is not alerted!

My Solution: _____

Obstacle 2. Eating for reasons other than nutrition

TDM Solution: Look for underlying limiting beliefs or out-of-date beliefs that no longer serve you but you have got into the habit of doing. Notice the behaviour and stop. Interrupt your pattern by removing yourself from the trigger point – go to the next room or outside. Choose another behaviour that you enjoy that will take your mind away from its old regular path down into a negative habit. Come up with another new belief or new habit that does serve you and practise repeating it and living it every time the situation arises. Match the solution to the trigger – if bored – find something you love to do and do that. If sad, ring a friend. If anxious or distracted, go for a walk in the fresh air and get calm.

My Solution: _____

Your new approach may mean the obstacles that you put on your list may not even seem like obstacles to you anymore. Once you see them as the pathway to personal growth taking you a step closer to your goal each time you overcome one, then you needn't approach them with such dread. They are more like challenges that teach you to grow as you find solutions. As you learn the tools and techniques to help you resolve them, then you know what to do when they come along next time.

Having a clear direction of where that finish line is will also help. For a good part of our lives, we just knew we wanted to lose weight but did not really either have the right motives or understood the value of having the right consistency of action. In a way, we were lost out there in diet land, going round and round in circles, being stopped by the same old obstacles and never moving forward. If you know where you are going, then you can bypass a few of them. You know which ones are the ones you need to go over, which ones you can go round and which ones to not worry so much about. Eventually you may even get to the place where you start to relish the challenge of being an overcomer!

You will learn what works for you and know that if you keep doing it consistently, day by day, you will get to where you want to go.

As somebody once said *"It won't happen overnight, but it will happen."*

Afterword

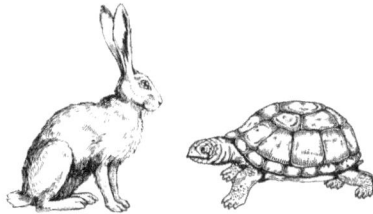

I hope this book does show you a way to go from where you thought you were supposed to go but could never get there - traditional diet land with its empty promises of miracle results - towards the much more achievable winning post of your personal vision for your life.

Thanks to this ancient fable, I came up with a completely different approach to the problem. It enabled me to walk away from the old model altogether which was such a relief because that one was overloaded with a lot of old baggage, beliefs, behaviours, and impossible deadlines. The miracle diet model could no longer be revived and was ready to be laid to rest.

So...here's a big shout out to our two heroes, the hare and tortoise. Even though I have spent most of the book pointing my finger at the hare as an example of what not to do, and how much we should be more like the tortoise, we are of course both the hare and the tortoise.

We all carry the potential of both. Our best results come when we integrate the two. Imagine the natural flare, talent and drive of the hare if it was combined with the steadiness, discipline and quiet determination of the tortoise.

My wish for you is that you discover and learn from the tortoise and the hare within you, overcome the pain of those old obstacles to finally win your own race and then make a lifelong habit of outrageous wellbeing and success.

References and Resources

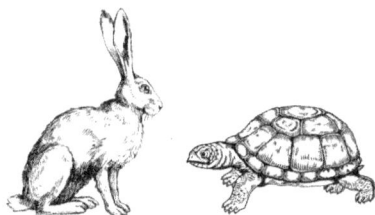

Pollan, Michael (2006) The Omnivores Dilemma
Weaver, Dr Libby (2010) Accidentally Overweight
Weaver, Dr Libby (2014) The Calorie Fallacy
Mosley, Dr Michael (2018) The Fast 800
Duhigg, Charles (2012) The Power of Habit
Spackman, Dr Kerry (2009) The Winner's Bible
Pressfield, Steven (2002) The War of Art

About the Author

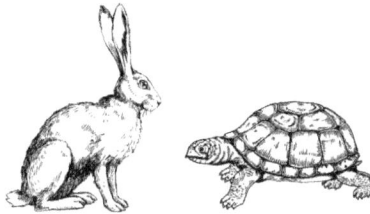

Keren Mackay comes from a rural New Zealand farming background and graduated from Auckland University with a BA in English and History. She has raised 3 children, untold chickens, lambs, ponies, dogs and any other animal (or child) that joined the queue in her farmhouse kitchen. She was a librarian for many years and later worked in events and hospitality before more recently spending more than a dozen years working as a Museum Professional.

Her side hustle, the Professional Countrywoman came as a direct result of watching herself and her friends juggling all the jobs that face the busy rural entrepreneur, managing households and tripping over gumboots at the back door while attempting to get themselves together for the next zoom call. When the time came to put her occupation on any form, the answer was clearly a "Professional Countrywoman!"

Her mission is to encourage women to care for their own wellbeing as they go about the vitally important business of raising the next generation, creating wealth and sharing it. Now that she has graduated to becoming a grandmother it's the next generation that has become her audience — she teaches workshops on how to grow food for the family, simple ways to preserve and prepare the food, and also reminding and encouraging women to care for themselves as they contribute to the health, wealth and wellbeing of the family.

Her book, the *Tortoise Diet Method*, is part of that wellbeing focus as she observed the often painful and pointless process of constantly battling with food and weight and how it occupied too much unnecessary headspace in not just her own head but in those around her. As you can imagine given her background, the book takes a sensible kitchen table approach to a genuine concern for women of all ages, but particularly as they get older and see the upward trajectory of the number on the scales with the attendant health problems.

Once she decided that she never wanted to go on a diet ever again, but still wanted to look and feel good, she found inspiration in the age-old tale of the Tortoise and the Hare. The Tortoise Diet Method provides the blueprint to successfully overcome years of diet failure by identifying and taking the time to deal with what has stopped us in the past and shows how to take the right steps slowly and steadily towards winning your race.

Keren is available for speaking or workshop engagements on the key messages from the book including topics such as

From failure to freedom – 5 steps to turn lifelong diet failure into fit and fabulous.

From food police to food peace; getting to the bottom of the disordered thinking behind serial diet failure.

Workshops.

Weekend workshops to go through the 12 Guideposts of success found in her book, the Tortoise Diet Method.

Practical ways to grow food for the family in the backyard vegetable patch, specialising in planning and planting calendars for crop rotation. Can be tailored to beginners.

You can contact Keren at www.professionalcountrywoman.com or www.tortoisedietmethod.com

Email: keren@professionalcountrywoman.com

Facebook: https://www.facebook.com/profile.php?id=100040489152798 or The Professional Countrywoman.

Or https://www.facebook.com/TortoiseDietMethod/

THE TORTOISE ~~DIET~~ *Method*

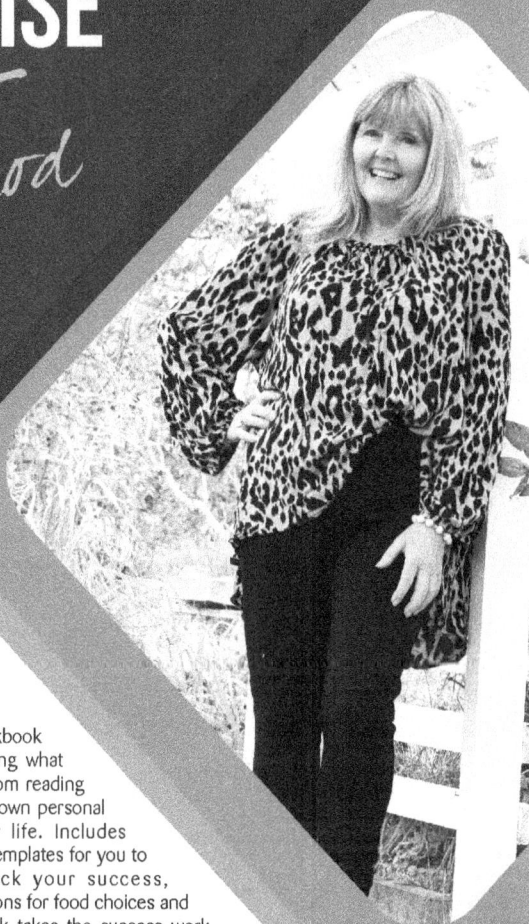

Facebook

Begin your journey by becoming part of the community on facebook. Join www.facebook.com/TortoiseDietMethod to enjoy being inspired and encouraged as well as keep up with any news.

Workbook

Download your FREE Tortoise Diet Method Workbook NOW to start turning what you have learned from reading this book into your own personal blueprint for your life. Includes graphs, tables and templates for you to measure and track your success, inspiration, suggestions for food choices and more. The workbook takes the success work from each chapter and puts it into a simple format for you to finally achieve success in the race to reach your own finish line.

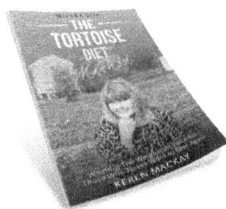

Your Tortoise Diet Method Workbook can be downloaded by going to this link: www.thetortoisedietmethod.com

Courses and Workshops

Now you have read the book and started to become hopeful about finding your own balanced and healthy bodyweight again, then you may need to have extra help and support. Find out more about what on-line courses or workshops you can join to help you get a firm foundation for future success.

From Tortoise Diet Lite – a short taster for those who are not sure if they really believe it is possible, through to a 12 week foundation course or the full 12 month ElevateElite course including private coaching, there will be a way that suits you at whatever stage of life you are in.

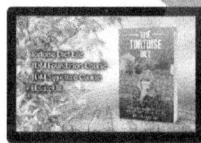

www.ingramcontent.com/pod-product-compliance
Lightning Source LLC
Chambersburg PA
CBHW022053020426
42335CB00012B/665